D0049425

ER NURSES

For a complete list of books by James Patterson, as well as previews of upcoming books and more information about the author, visit JamesPatterson.com or find him on Facebook.

ER NURSES

True Stories from America's Greatest Unsung Heroes

James Patterson
and Matt Eversmann
with Chris Mooney

Little, Brown and Company

New York Boston London

Copyright © 2021 by James Patterson

Little, Brown and Company
Hachette Book Group
1290 Avenue of the Americas, New York, NY 10104
littlebrown.com

First Edition: October 2021

Little, Brown and Company is a division of Hachette Book Group, Inc. The Little, Brown name and logo are trademarks of Hachette Book Group, Inc.

The publisher is not responsible for websites (or their content) that are not owned by the publisher.

The Hachette Speakers Bureau provides a wide range of authors for speaking events. To find out more, go to hachettespeakersbureau.com or call (866) 376-6591.

ISBN 978-0-759-55426-9 (hardcover) / 978-0-316-30107-7 (large print)
LCCN 2021931657

10 9 8 7 6 5 4 3 2 1

MRQ-T

Printed in Canada

To Nancy Stine Eversmann

CONTENTS

CONTENTS

PART ONE:

Day Shift

ANGELA PARAWAN

Angela Parawan was born in New York City and grew up in Virginia Beach. After graduating from nursing school, she did an externship at a cardiovascular ICU. Angela is a traveling nurse and currently lives in California.

I don't think I'm cut out to be a nurse.

Growing up, I watched my mother take good care of my extended family, especially my grandmother. My interest in becoming a professional caregiver sparked, I toyed with the idea of becoming a doctor—until I shadowed one and found out how little time doctors spend with patients.

And I want the human interactions, so I chose nursing.

But nursing school, I'm finding, is hard. I'm struggling with the dual responsibilities of attending class during the day and working as a nursing assistant at night.

The hospital job is important because it's a front-row seat to the reality of nursing. The nurses here run around at a hundred miles a minute, all the while projecting to everyone that they are cool, calm, and collected.

I admire their composure, because I'm an empath. I'm highly sensitive to what other people are thinking and feeling. I take on their emotions, their pain. A lot of the nurses here share that trait. They have more heart than they let on.

And then there's death. It comes in waves, and lately we've had a lot. When someone dies, it *really* affects me, and it really affects the other nurses too because, deep down, like me, they're nurturers. But they can't show it. They have to be rational, steady, fully in control of their emotions.

There's no way I can do this for a career, I think as a nurse delivers a new patient to one of the open rooms on our floor.

His name is Brian. His wife is with him. They both look shell-shocked.

"I came into the hospital tonight because I'm not feeling well," Brian explains as the nurse and I get him settled. "I was holding a lot of fluid in my stomach, and I wanted to see what's what. They ran a couple of tests, and it's...I have pancreatic cancer."

Brian is a professor at one of the colleges. He's a super-nice guy, former navy, and really, really accomplished. He's so kind to the staff—so thankful. The staff love him. I love him. We gravitate toward him because of his demeanor, how he handles himself as he tries to fight the disease.

One night, as I'm talking with Brian, I share my struggles with him.

"You can do this," he tells me. "Going to school during the day, working nights—I know it's hard. It's supposed to be. Remember, nothing that's worthwhile in life comes easy."

I come from a family of nurses and doctors. They've essentially given me the same advice—to hang in there, be resilient. They're supportive because they're my family. But the conviction in Brian's words and the confident way he says them leaves an indelible impression on me.

In the two months he's with us, I watch his physical abilities decline. He can no longer walk, can't even stand up or roll over in bed.

"We've been married for forty-five years," his wife tells me. "I don't know what I'm going to do without him—I don't even know who I'll be without him."

Brian's death hits me hard. I cling to his words as I continue my struggle through nursing school. I think of him when I graduate.

At twenty-five years old, I'm a traveling nurse. Every three months, I get to pick where I'd like to work. I've decided to finish up my stint in Colorado Springs, take a month off, then move to New York City. My family spent many summers there when I was young, and I enjoyed those times, but I've never been there as an adult.

I arrive in early March of 2020. The first two weeks are fun. I work three days a week and explore the city on my days off.

I'm aware of COVID. It's on my radar, but it hasn't hit NYC yet.

The travel company I'm working for calls me and says, "The hospital is going to transition you into overflow."

During cold and flu season, hospitals can get overcrowded, so they often have designated areas to deal with a high volume of sick patients. On top of that, my hospital is also expecting an influx of COVID patients.

"Be prepared to work forty-eight to seventy-two hours each week."

"Okay," I say, wondering if I'm going to get an N95 mask and proper protective equipment. "Will do."

The hospital gives us each a simple surgical mask. Because of the limited supply, the mask when not in use is to be stored in a brown paper bag and then reused until it's soiled. Because I'll be working in the COVID unit and the COVID ICU, I can wear my gown multiple times. When it's soiled, I'll be given another one.

We're each given a respirator (a mask with a filter) in a bag labeled with our name. Respirators are designed to be used once and for no longer than one hour. But now, as long as they're not soiled, we're to reuse them until they fall apart.

COVID hits New York fast and hard. The hospital insists we wear our masks continuously throughout our twelve-hour shifts. The constant wear causes blisters on my nose and my cheeks. My skin breaks down. One day after work, when I take off my mask, the skin peels off my nose. It just rips right off.

During a thirteen- to fourteen-hour day, carbon dioxide builds up inside the masks. The gas is unsafe in high concentration. A couple of nurses on my floor pass out from inhaling too much CO_2.

I use the respirator I'm given for three weeks.

By April, the COVID cases have risen alarmingly. One day, we have close to eleven thousand cases.

If I don't have COVID now, I think, *I'm going to get it.*

The majority of our patients who need to be intubated don't ever make it out of the hospital.

Some days, instead of working in the COVID ICU, I'm floated to other floors with COVID patients who need lower levels of care. It's there I get word that one of my ICU COVID patients has been taken off the ventilator and is breathing on his own. He's being transferred to me.

His voice is really raspy, and he's still very weak and very, very sick. He shouldn't be alive—I was sure he was going to die. He may very well still die.

This guy not only survives, but in a couple of weeks he's up and walking. Healthy. When he leaves our hospital, people line up in the hallways to cheer him on. He's the first patient who's gotten off the vent and made it out of here.

One day I have five patients, all young guys. Four of them die.

It's one of the most horrific things I've ever seen. I've never had so many patients die in one day. It's the worst thing emotionally that's ever happened to me. When I leave the hospital at nine p.m., I'm physically and mentally exhausted. I've got nothing left.

I live a mile away and walk home every night. This area was, not that long ago, very busy and had high foot traffic. Now it's completely empty except for homeless people. And rats, which are at an all-time high. They're everywhere you look.

The emptiness of the streets...it's such an eerie feeling. Stores are open, their lights on, but there are only a few people around. When they see me dressed in my scrubs, they turn away or move to the opposite side of the street because they know I work at the hospital and they think I'm probably infected with COVID.

Usually, I feel proud to be a nurse. Now I feel like a leper.

When I get home, the stress I've been under these past six weeks—waking up at four every day to go to work, the long, grueling hours, the deaths, the suffering and trauma—all of it finally takes its toll. I call my mom and tell her what's happening.

"Are you okay?" she asks.

"This is so much harder than I expected." Then I lose it. I start crying hysterically. "I don't think I can do this. All of my patients are dying—I can't handle it anymore, Mom. If I catch COVID and I'm on a vent, please just let me go."

My mom listens patiently and does her best to console me.

"A lot of nurses are just up and leaving New York," I tell her. "They don't even show up for work. Today, I was supposed to be working with a guy named Paul. I couldn't find him, and when I asked where he was, I was told, 'Oh, he's not coming in. He's on a plane right now going back to wherever he's from.'"

"Can they actually do that? Isn't that—what do you call it again?"

"Abandonment. In any other time, yes, it would be reported to the board of nursing. But this is COVID, so they're ignoring it because when someone leaves, the hospital has another warm body who is willing to fill that spot almost instantly. There are so many nurses flooding into the city to help."

"Do you want to leave? Come home?"

A part of me does. Of course a part of me does. Who wouldn't want to get away from this stress, exhaustion, and death?

Then I recall Brian's words: *I know it's hard. It's supposed to be. Remember, nothing that's worthwhile in life comes easy.*

I'm doing something others can't. I'm still here, and I'm able to hold my head high because I know who I am, and I'm not a quitter. Running away isn't an option.

My years in nursing have taught me resiliency. I've stayed the course through uncomfortable situations that had me questioning who I was, doubting my skills as a nurse. Each time, I emerged on the other side stronger from my experience—stronger mentally, physically, and emotionally.

I will handle this pandemic because I can handle more than I give myself credit for. I'm a nurse. I can handle anything.

KATIE QUICK

Katie Quick lives in Virginia. She worked on the medical-surgical floors and in the ICU before becoming an emergency department nurse.

The older man lying in the ICU bed is dying. I don't think he's even aware that he's surrounded by his family—his wife and two adult sons.

"Is there anything I can do for you?" I ask them. "For him?"

The wife dabs her face with a tissue. "All he'd want is his dog."

"Go home and get him."

The family turns to me.

"What?" the wife asks.

"Go home and bring the dog here."

I'm pretty new in my ICU career, and though I suspect bringing a dog here is against hospital policy, I don't care. If my dad were dying, he would want his dog. (This was long before therapy animals became an actual thing.)

The sons return with the dog—a golden retriever. It's three o'clock in the morning. I sneak the dog up the back hallway. Because the man's bed is pretty high, I help lift the retriever up. The dog snuggles up to the man and rests its head under the guy's arm.

The dog stays with him all night long.

The hospital administrators aren't pleased. I get called on the carpet, but I don't care. The patient was dying. The family said he needed his dog, and I made sure that happened.

My most memorable moment in the ICU involves a married couple.

The man is pretty young—in his forties—and he's a home-hospice patient dying of cancer. Home-hospice patients have a team in place that helps them deal with pain, anxiety, and malnutrition, and death is usually imminent.

Once a hospice patient calls 911 or comes into the ED, he or she becomes a patient seeking treatment. The man's wife said she wanted his code status reversed, which means we have to do whatever we can to keep him alive.

"I just couldn't let him die at home," the wife tells me. "We have two young kids."

Her husband is not verbally responsive at this point. His blood pressure is very low, so we've put him on IV medication. He's also on oxygen because he needs a lot of respiratory support.

There's no question he's going to die. It's just a matter of when.

My mother refused to take her kids to funerals because she didn't want to expose us to that level of sadness. There's no escaping it in the ICU—and that's not the only place you find it.

My last semester of nursing school, I did a clinical rotation in a nursing home where you're assigned one patient and you spend the whole day with them. I took one lady to her activity, then brought her back, got her cleaned up, put her in bed, and went to my noon conference. When I checked on her afterward, I discovered that she had passed.

I cried and cried—I could not get it together. The family had to console *me*. They rubbed my back and told me, "It's okay, honey. We knew she was going to pass."

I was twenty years old and hadn't had any experience with death and dying.

I went home that night thinking, *If I can't deal with a ninety-year-old dying, there is no way I can work with sick babies in the neonatal ICU.* I decided to reroute my career and went to work on a medical-surgical floor—with a large elderly population.

I've got to get a handle on the experience of death, I told myself. *I have to figure out how to better help families going through the transition of their loved ones.*

And I want to help this woman deal with her husband's eventual death in the ICU. I can tell she's at her wit's end even before she says, "I'm not ready for this."

I understand how she feels.

When I was a new ICU nurse, my brother-in-law was in a horrible motorcycle accident and had to be flown to a trauma center. The medevac providers couldn't do much, but they kept him alive, and what they gave me and my family was time. Time to sit with him, time to be with him and love him until a priest gave him the last rites. I got to be there with all of them to make sure he was treated with dignity and to watch him pass.

I'm about to speak when her husband soils himself.

In a situation like this, I typically tell the family member to step outside, go to the cafeteria. But for some reason, I say, "I'm going to clean him up. Do you want to help?"

She looks at me with the most incredulous expression, one that says, *Are you serious?*

"He's your husband," I say. "You can help me if you want, or you can leave the room."

She starts crying. "I've been his caretaker, giving him his medications and tube feedings, but I haven't seen him naked in six months. He's been afraid to show me his body because he's so skinny."

"Let me get everything we'll need, and we'll do it together."

As we wash and clean her husband, it's clear how physically and emotionally spent she is. We talk about all sorts of stuff, and as she rubs his back and then massages his feet, she confesses she hasn't had sex with him for over a year and a half. Washing him and cleaning his bottom is the most intimate she's been with him since he got sick.

Looking at her face, I can see just how much in love she is with her husband, even under the gross and cruel circumstances.

After I clean up and take out the trash, I say, "I want your husband to rest right now. How about you? Do you need to rest?"

"I'm exhausted."

I put his bedrail down and pull back his covers. "Would you like to take a nap with him?"

She starts crying and crying and crying.

"Can I?" she asks.

"Of course. He's your husband."

"We haven't slept in the same bed for six months."

She climbs in. I turn down the lights and put on some soft music.

Some of my older coworkers aren't happy about what I've done. One nurse begins to approach me.

I've lost count of the number of times a nurse or doctor has said, "Put the family in the waiting room." I want to scream, *Bullshit*. Instead, I go get the family members, bring them to the bedside, and say, "Look at that monitor. See that right there? That's a heartbeat. There's life, so take this moment and take this time."

The nurse looks at me sternly now. "Katie, family members are not supposed to be in the bed with the patients."

"I didn't read that policy."

She's not happy with my flippant response. I don't care. I'm not like most nurses. I tell it like it is. Not everyone can be compassionate. It's not their fault. They're just programmed differently. Some people just aren't as sensitive as others. Some people aren't as emotional. As my mother told us growing up, some people need love the most when they least deserve it.

"He's her husband, and he's dying," I tell the older nurse. "Just leave them be."

The couple naps for four hours.

Her husband passes that night.

I truly believe I gave that woman the most amazing experience, one that she will always cherish. It's not something I signed up to do; I did it because it was right. I don't think people realize the fight that goes on in nurses' hearts—sticking to a hospital's legal policy versus acting on humanitarian impulses.

I will stand there with you and cry with you. I will print off a strip from the monitor that shows your loved one's heart was still beating while you were there, talking, holding a hand, giving a kiss.

AMBER RICHARDSON

Amber Richardson lives in Dallas, Texas, and works in an emergency department.

Nurses are at the center of it all.

Nurses are the first ones to see a patient. We take your vitals, assess the situation, and initiate the orders—start your IV, your labs—before you see the doctor. And you see the doctor for only a few minutes; a nurse is constantly monitoring you. When a doctor orders the wrong medication or the wrong dose, we're the ones who catch the errors. I don't think the general public knows just how much nurses do.

The Hispanic man who comes into the ER is young, in his mid-thirties, and somewhat overweight. His name is Daniel, and around his neck he's wearing a rosary with a crucifix. He says he's having abdominal pain that's radiating to his back.

I ask him about his medical history. He says he doesn't have one.

"I don't ever need to go to the doctor," Daniel says.

Which doesn't surprise me. I've learned from experience that most Hispanic men rarely, if ever, get yearly check-ups. They also rarely complain when they're hurting. They're workaholics, driven to provide for their families. When a Hispanic man comes into the ER and says he's in pain, we tend to take him seriously.

The man's wife and nine-year-old son accompany him to the exam room. The other nurses and I hook Daniel up to the monitor and, because he's dehydrated, get an IV started.

I have this weird feeling that something's not right. I order a CT scan.

Daniel's family stays in the room while I take him up to get the scan. When we return, they're gone. I get a call from the radiologist, who confirms my suspicions about Daniel.

"Your patient has an abdominal aortic aneurysm that's about to rupture. He needs to go to surgery *right now*."

Because if it ruptures, he could die.

As I explain this to Daniel and let him know what will happen next, my gut tells me that I need to find his family and bring them back here before he goes into surgery because it might be the last time his wife and son will see him alive. His family needs to be here to say goodbye.

I find out they went to the cafeteria. I run down there, get them, and bring them back to the room. A doctor is there. He explains why Daniel needs emergency surgery.

The wife is visibly struggling as she realizes the severity of her husband's condition. Tears are flowing down her face, and the nine-year-old, who's standing there watching and listening, is absolutely terrified.

"Okay," I tell Daniel, "you need to give your family a hug. We've got to take you to surgery."

Daniel slowly takes off his rosary beads and places them around his son's neck. We wheel him away to surgery.

It doesn't go well. Daniel codes. He's brought to the ICU. A few days later, he dies.

While the outcome hurts, I find some solace in the fact that I made sure Daniel saw his family. Daniel being able to hand over the rosary to his son—that will be the boy's last memory of his father.

Working in the ER, you see people die all the time. You learn the ideal way you want to die. One patient I have is a man in his sixties. He has terminal cancer and a host of medical complications, and when he comes into the ER, he's barely coherent.

He's surrounded by his three daughters, all grown women in their forties. They've decided not to allow any further treatment or CPR if he codes. They want their father to pass peacefully.

I bring in chairs so they can sit with him.

"Your dad isn't really aware of what's going on, but he can hear you," I tell them. "The thing he would want most right now would be for y'all to share stories from when you were kids and to just laugh and have fun with that."

As I make my rounds, I hear these women laughing and telling these amazing stories, and it makes me smile. I want to stop working and go in there and join them.

I truly believe this father knows his girls are with him. Being surrounded by my children as they laugh and giggle and tell stories and share fond memories from their childhood—that, for me, would be the best way to die.

ANDREA PERRY

Andrea Perry followed her mom and her aunt into nursing. She is a staff nurse in an emergency department on the West Coast.

An ER tech is pushing a young woman in a wheelchair. The patient is completely unresponsive, barely breathing. I move to the wheelchair, locate the portable monitor the tech has placed her on, and lean in to look at the readings.

The woman's heart rate is high, her oxygen dangerously low.

"Boyfriend thinks she accidentally overdosed on some pain medication," the tech tells me. "She recently underwent plastic surgery—breast augmentation."

"How old is she?"

"Twenty-three."

Oh my God, this girl is a year younger than me.

"The boyfriend kept waiting for her to wake up. Two hours passed, and when she didn't come out of it, Mr. Wonderful thought it would be a fantastic idea to drive her here instead of calling 911."

We exchange a look, both of us thinking the same thing: *Something fishy is going on.* Maybe the two of them were into some shady stuff and he didn't want the police to find out.

That's not my problem. My focus is on saving this woman's life.

Normally, I'd bring a patient in critical condition to the area we call the front wall—one of our larger rooms that holds one to two patients. Those beds are currently full, but I have an open treatment room. It will be tight quarters, but we don't have a choice.

Our ER doctor and nurses swarm over this young woman, whose name is Cindy. We quickly strip off her clothes and intubate her. I have someone call the pharmacy.

"Where's the boyfriend?" I ask, searching for a vein on the woman's arm to start an IV. "The waiting room?"

"He's gone," the tech replies. "He didn't stick around."

The collection area inside the breathing tube, I notice, has pink, frothy sputum, an indication that fluid has collected inside her lungs.

My thoughts turn to ARDS, or acute respiratory distress syndrome. Right now, her body is shutting down because the fluid in her lungs is preventing oxygen from getting into her bloodstream.

"Call RT!" I shout. Respiratory therapy needs to suction the woman's breathing tube.

After we intubate someone, we often see a positive response in the patient's vital signs. Cindy's are still poor. She's going to need multiple medications to raise her blood pressure, slow down her heart rate, and prevent the continued collection of fluid in her lungs. The drugs can't be mixed together, and they need to be given intravenously.

Only we can't find a single vein anywhere on her extremities or her neck.

We can't give Cindy her meds and fluids without IV access, so she needs a central line. A central line is inserted into a large vein, usually in the chest area, and only a doctor can do the procedure.

Dr. Baker, the ER doc who initially treated Cindy, has left to see other patients. I rush off to find him.

"She doesn't need a central line," Dr. Baker tells me. "It's just an OD. The drugs will wear off. Keep trying to find a peripheral vein."

I go back to the patient and try to find a peripheral vein.

I can't. Something needs to be done right now or Cindy might very well die.

The general message you receive as a nurse, through schooling and in your career, is to do what you're told. I'm a young nurse. A part of me says, *Well, the doctor doesn't think the patient needs a central line, so I'll listen to him.* My job, though, is to take care of the patient, and that also means advocating for the patient.

Dr. Baker made it clear he doesn't think my patient needs a central line. As much as I'd like to find another doctor to do the procedure for me, I have to respect the chain of command.

I find Dr. Baker in the room where doctors do their charts and dictations. He's not alone. Four other doctors are with him.

Maybe I can use them as leverage. I quickly come up with a plan.

"Who wants to help me save my patient's life?" I ask the room.

The doctors—especially Baker—all look at me.

"I have a patient in bed six who has ARDS," I say. "She's dying. Can one of you help me save her by putting in a central line?"

Baker gets up, doing his best to hide his embarrassment at the public shaming. He doesn't speak as he accompanies me back to Cindy's bed. He's probably angry at me, and that's okay. I have a good reputation, and I'm fighting for the best interests of my patient.

He puts in a central line. An ICU doctor arrives and orders some medications to raise Cindy's blood pressure. We get her on at least three IV drips. We manage to stabilize her and remove the fluid from her lungs.

Cindy is a thin woman. When I see her the next day, I barely recognize her—she's so puffed out from all the fluids we've given her that she looks like the Marshmallow Man. Her CT scan shows cerebral edema and some other serious signs that explain her decreased level of consciousness.

A doctor has noted on Cindy's chart that her chance of survival is 20 percent.

I'm crushed by the note. I fought so hard for her. I so badly wanted a better outcome.

Still, it's early days. I refuse to give up hope.

The boyfriend never shows up, but the mother does. Once. She does not seem concerned at all for her daughter; in fact, she appears rather put out by the whole experience. She leaves as soon as possible.

One day, I go to check on Cindy, and I'm surprised—and happy—to see two women in her room, looking at their phones. *Must be her friends*, I think. They're roughly the same age as Cindy.

These two women start taking pictures of Cindy. One giggles quietly. When I enter the room, I see the other one posting a picture of Cindy on her social media account.

I want to rip into them. *What's wrong with you two? This woman nearly died, she's unconscious, and she's most likely going to be a vegetable—what kind of person thinks it's funny to come in here, take pictures of a friend in such a vulnerable state, and post them for the entire world to see? You're sick. You both make me sick.*

I remind myself to remain professional. Still, my anger and disgust come through loud and clear when I say, "Taking photos of a patient without her consent is unacceptable. You're going to delete those photos right now and remove them from all your social media accounts."

I watch them to make sure they do as they're told. When the photos have been taken down and deleted, I have security escort the two women out of the hospital.

I'm shaken and horrified—for Cindy. Her boyfriend has disappeared, her mom can't be bothered—and these two women are her *friends*?

Does she have anyone in her life who loves her? Cares for her in any way? Did this poor woman ever have a shot at a good and decent life?

I feel sick to my stomach. I break down in tears.

Days turn into weeks. Cindy's condition is stable, but poor. She's still unconscious. Intubated.

One day I come to work, check the ICU board, and find out that Cindy's name is missing. She's been moved to the telemetry unit, a lower level of care but one where her internal functions and vital signs can still be constantly monitored.

I know the harsh reality of Cindy's condition. I figure she

still can't breathe on her own, but you can't be intubated long term, so the solution is a tracheostomy. Doctors have made an incision in the trachea to create a stoma, or hole, wide enough for a tube through which she can be ventilated.

I assume a decision has already been made to transfer Cindy to a long-term-care facility.

My heart breaks—and not because she's my patient. This poor young woman doesn't have a single positive person in her life. Her mother and boyfriend don't care about her—no one does.

Except me. I head to telemetry to let her know I care about her. To say goodbye.

"I was Cindy's nurse in the ER," I tell one of the telemetry nurses. "Is it okay if I pop in?"

The nurse nods. "Today's her birthday."

That hits me even harder. *Now we're the exact same age.*

I walk into the room and find Cindy sitting cross-legged on the bed, flipping through the TV channels.

I start crying. Cindy looks at me, confused.

"It's good to see you doing so well," I say. "Happy birthday."

Cindy smiles. "Thank you."

I wipe at my eyes. "You probably don't remember me, but I took care of you in the emergency room."

"I remember you. Thank you so much."

I don't know if that's true. She was so out of it when I saw her.

But it doesn't matter. I'm simply overjoyed she's alive, this person who had only a 20 percent chance of survival.

I did the right thing, fighting for her. I knew what my patient needed. I fought for her, and I didn't give up.

That's what nursing is about.

CAROL RICE

Carol Rice entered the order of the Adrian Dominican Sisters with the intention of becoming a nun. Two and a half years later, she took an EMT class that led to her to become an ER nurse. Carol recently retired and now lives in South Haven, Michigan.

Working at Detroit Receiving is the Wild West of nursing, and the cases are pretty extreme.

Like this man they just brought in. Both of his legs have been amputated—by a train. He owed money to his bookie, so the bookie had some guys hold him down on a railroad track until a train came.

He's still alive, and the stumps aren't bleeding much because they're "traumatically sealed." As he's rushed down the hall to the OR, someone shouts to me: *"Hey, Rice, get the legs."*

For a moment, I'm puzzled. Then I'm told another ambulance has just arrived with the legs.

I've been working in the ER since Detroit Receiving opened

in 1980. I started as an EMT and then went to school to become a nurse. That first year, we saw over a hundred thousand patients, a good majority of them suffering from penetrating trauma—wounds created by weapons and other sharp objects. The hospital quickly earned the nickname "the Knife and Gun Club."

The pace in the ER is extremely fast. Crazy and wild. I discovered that I was really good with my hands and I could think clearly under pressure. Working here suits my need for constant variety. To me, there's nothing worse than seeing the same people every day, and there's no chance of that happening here.

Both of the man's severed legs are still covered in the torn brown fabric of his pants. A brown sock is on one foot. I can't carry both of the legs—they're too heavy—so I rush them down one leg at a time.

The man ends up bleeding out and dying. His legs are put on the specimen table to be transferred to pathology. For some reason, they're left on the table all weekend, and come Monday, the decomposing legs have stunk up the whole place.

My next patient is withdrawing from alcohol and has the DTs. I put him in a chair about five feet away from where I'm working so I can keep an eye on him. He has hair like Don King—it's waxed and stands up straight. He's in two-point restraints so he can't go anywhere, but that doesn't keep him from talking to every person who walks past him.

"Can I get a cigarette?" he asks. "Anybody got a cigarette?"

It's the early 1980s; smoking is allowed in hospitals. I decide to give him a cigarette, thinking that if I just let him hold it, maybe the unlit cigarette might help him relax.

An ER patient in the trauma module—he's not one of mine—grabs me and says, "I'm in so much pain. Can someone please help me?"

I go check with his nurse, a woman everyone here admires—she's the top cop in the ER, and she's become sort of a personal hero of mine. I see the care and compassion she gives her patients, and because I'm still relatively new to nursing, I've tried to model her behavior.

She tells me she's already given him Demerol. After I check in on my patient in the trauma module, I head back to the nurses' station. I'm there working when I smell smoke.

I turn around and see the guy going through the DTs has a cone of flame on top of his head. Someone lit the cigarette I gave him and now his hair is on fire.

A tech and I grab blankets to put out the fire. The man is okay, but his hair is now much, much shorter.

I go back to the trauma module, and the man I saw earlier—the one who was in so much pain—is now in tears. He grabs my arm again and says, "I'm in terrible pain. *Please, please help me.*"

It turns out his nurse wasn't giving him Demerol. She was injecting him with saline and taking the Demerol herself. We find her passed out in the bathroom.

Suddenly, certain things I've seen and certain things she's done make sense—the fact that she always has small pupils; how every morning she hands me a list of things to do and then disappears for a good half an hour.

It's an eye-opening experience, one that also leaves me feeling disillusioned.

I started smoking at sixteen and quit when I was twenty-one.

There are so many times when the pressure in my neck is so bad that I feel like my head is going to explode, but instead of smoking, to deal with stress, I run with my partner—a high-school teacher who is a really steady person—for about an hour every evening. We talk about our days. I get the first half an hour; she gets the second.

Detroit Receiving is really crazy, and the trauma I see is violent and continuous. One day I ask myself, *What's a nice girl like you doing in a place like this?*

I love working in the ER. After sixteen years at Detroit Receiving, I decide to take a job in the ER at a suburban hospital.

I'm sitting behind a Plexiglas barrier triaging a patient with chest pain when a man who looks like Santa Claus comes up to me and says, in a very polite voice, "Can I talk to you?"

"I'm busy with a patient right now. I'll be with you in a moment."

"Oh, I'm so sorry."

He reaches over the top of the Plexiglas barrier and drops a note. In my mind, the note seems to be falling through the air in slow motion, like it's floating. Before the note hits the floor, I see the word *Kevorkian*.

Oh my gosh.

It's 1990 and Dr. Kevorkian, a pathologist, has started helping people who are suffering from terminal illnesses end their lives. He's all over the news because he's been dropping bodies off at ERs in different local hospitals.

And now it looks like he might possibly be here at mine.

I don't pick up the note. I look to one of the other nurses and say, "Finish this triage."

Outside, police are swarming around Kevorkian's "death van"—an old, beat-up white Volkswagen van pockmarked with rust. It's parked right near the emergency entrance.

The van's side door is open. A big guy is sitting slumped over in his seat. He's clearly dead.

The police rush in front of me. "Don't touch anything. This is a crime scene!"

Santa Claus Guy (who I'll later find out is Kevorkian's assistant) is talking to the police. My attention is on the small older man standing next to the van's open door.

Dr. Kevorkian.

The charge nurse enters the fracas. She looks at me and says, "Bring that patient in here right now. We're going to resuscitate him."

Our hospital has implemented what's called the Kevorkian protocol. If the man drives his van up to our hospital, we treat his passenger as we would any patient.

I push a stretcher up to the van and step inside. The male slumped against the seat weighs, I'm guessing, at least two hundred fifty pounds. As I grip him underneath the arms, Kevorkian says, "Don't you do that, he's too big for you."

Kevorkian moves around to the other side of the van and opens the door. He pushes the man and I pull until I'm finally able to load him onto the stretcher.

The whole scene—a van pulling up to an ER with a dead body, the staff performing CPR on that dead body—is grim. What's even grimmer to me is that I don't disagree with Kevorkian.

As a nurse, I've dealt with patients who are suffering with terminal diseases and others who have such serious, complicated medical problems that they have no quality of life. If these people want to die, it should be their decision.

Kevorkian is doing publicly what ICU doctors here at the hospital have done privately. Kevorkian is making a statement—one that is now getting national headlines—that terminal patients should be allowed to choose when to end their lives.

In the following months, Dr. Kevorkian continues to drop off bodies at various Michigan hospitals. But then he gets a little kooky. Before he delivers one man's body to an ER, he takes out the patient's kidneys. He lets doctors know the kidneys are available for transplant. But they can't be used because they were removed in an unsterile environment and not properly tested.

It's the beginning of his downfall. Shortly thereafter, he's arrested.

Dr. Kevorkian's methods—and the news he generates—causes a ripple effect through the medical community.

One of my patients suffers a massive stroke. She's not going to have a good outcome. One resident doctor writes an order for me to give this patient 20 milligrams of morphine—enough to kill an elephant.

"I can't give that," I tell the resident. "That's not an emergency order—and I'm not Dr. Kevorkian."

I bring the order to the attending physician, who is shocked and horrified. Sometimes I feel that nurses are the only safeguard preventing bad things from happening at the hospital.

After working in this ER for nineteen years, I decide I've

had enough. I've already seen too many things that people should never see. I retire.

I take some time off and then decide to volunteer with the Red Cross. When a hurricane rips through North Carolina and causes massive flooding, I work with displaced residents who are sheltered at a local high school. When they are moved to a storeroom at the local Piggly Wiggly, I go with them. When wildfires ravage California, I go there, and I'm put in charge of a 265-patient shelter.

Some days, I really miss the ER. I don't miss the physically grueling twelve-hour shifts, but I miss the coworkers who became my family. I miss the Christmas songs I wrote for our parties. I miss the laughter and the camaraderie and the energy—and the good I did. The difference I made in some people's lives. I think I miss that most of all.

CLAYTON ROELLE

Clayton Roelle lives in Canton, Georgia, and works in the emergency department.

I've just finished my thirty-minute lunch break when my phone rings. The caller is Tracy, my preceptor, or teacher, here at the hospital where I'm doing my externship in the emergency department.

"Clay," she says, "there's a code heading to room ten."

I take off running. In the week I've been working here, nothing too serious has come into the ER.

I've never seen a code before—never seen anyone die.

I'd spent some time in the ED (the emergency department, which is the same thing as the emergency room, just a more modern term) during my second semester of nursing school. I was amazed at how well the nurses and doctors worked under intense pressure, how they responded to a crisis instead of reacting to it.

My adrenaline is already pumping as I reach the door. *This is it. This is where I get to show these people what I'm made of. This is where I prove I have what it takes to be here.*

The patient is a male who has been in a car accident. He was intubated in the field. Glass shards are embedded in his face, and he's bleeding from his mouth. He has a neck injury, but dealing with that will have to wait because he's in cardiac arrest, no circulation at all.

Tracy throws me a pair of gloves and says, "Get over to the table and start doing chest compressions."

I've never done chest compressions on an actual patient. Plenty on twenty-pound mannequins, sure, but never on an actual patient. Working on a human is not as clean as working on a mannequin—a lesson I quickly learned when I had to put a Foley catheter in a four-hundred-pound bedridden male covered in diarrhea. There's a huge difference between training versus reality.

I stand at the side of the table, on the patient's right. Everything I've learned in school comes crashing down inside my mind. For a moment, I freeze, unsure of what I'm supposed to do.

"Pump his chest," Tracy says.

I'm a former football player, and I've got a pretty decent build. I start pumping the man's chest hard. Two minutes ago, I was eating a turkey wrap. Now I'm face-to-face with a man who is essentially dead.

"Good compressions," says one of the doctors. "Keep it up."

I've got my feet underneath me now. I'm pumping so hard the table is shaking.

They finally get a pulse. The doctor makes an incision in the patient's chest so he can put in a chest tube, and blood shoots several feet in the air, splattering the walls and the floor.

When we get him stabilized, I leave the room. Tracy follows.

"Are you all right?" she asks.

"Yeah, I'm fine." But my mind hasn't had a chance to digest what just happened.

And Tracy senses that. "Okay," she says. "What tasks do you have to do right now?"

I know she's trying to redirect my focus to the other patients under my care.

"There's...I have to collect a urine sample in room eighteen," I say.

"Okay. Go do it."

After I collect the urine sample, I deal with another patient. He's angry at me because I forgot to bring him a blanket but he has no idea why I'm distracted.

It's more than that. My mind feels torn. One part of my brain is focused on the present, what I need to do next, while the other part is still processing the shock of what I've just seen, the chaos. Adrenaline is still surging through my veins.

To cope with the stress in my job, I start every morning the same way. I get on my knees and pray to God, thank Him for the opportunity to do His will. Then I hit the gym, shower, and go to work. I know I'm heading into a dogfight, but no matter what happens in the ER, my morning routine allows me to maintain consistency.

If I don't bring the punch, I'll get punched—physically, mentally, and emotionally. When I bring my best, then my job can't get the best of me.

Over time, I learn how to distance myself from traumatic events so I can focus on my job, my next task. When I see people die, I put the loss in the mental equivalent of a shoebox. The rough compartmentalization is probably not the healthiest habit, but it's the only option that keeps me functioning.

Sometimes my emotions do slip through.

My patient is in his seventies and has throat cancer. He's a rough country dude who can barely talk. He's not critical, but his disease has advanced to the point where he's going to be put on comfort care.

His wife is with him. "We met in high school when we were eighteen," she tells me. "Now we're both seventy-plus."

This rough old man wakes up, but he's super-groggy. "I don't know why you're still here," he says to her. It's difficult for him to talk, and I have to listen carefully to his words. "Just let me die. We've had a good life."

"If you're going to go," she says, "I'm going to be here with you."

Their exchange is so pure, and so uncommon. I don't see deep love from people, and I haven't experienced it myself, this "Well, if the world catches fire, we're just going to burn together." It's very cool to be in this moment with them, and the experience fills me with emotion. And hope.

SHANNEN KANE

Shannen Kane started in the emergency department as a new nursing-school graduate. She works as an ER nurse in North Carolina.

All the scrubs in the emergency department are color-coded. As a nursing assistant, I wore maroon scrubs. Now that I'm a nurse, I walk in on my first day wearing Carolina blue scrubs, and all I can think is *Oh my gosh, is this real life?*

I remind myself that I need to shift my thinking. When I was a nursing assistant dealing with patients, I would say, "I'll go get your nurse," or "I'll go tell your nurse." Now *I'm* the nurse.

I feel like I'm in an alternate universe.

Today is the start of my six-month orientation. I'm assigned what's called a preceptor—an experienced nurse who will be teaching and supervising me during clinical practice. Her name is Linda, and she is one of the charge nurses.

One of the big distinctions I'll have to learn to make among patients is sick versus not sick. It's that straightforward.

A man comes through the front doors. He's accompanied by his wife. He goes to triage, and from there he's brought to one of our main trauma bays.

When I look at this patient, I see he's diaphoretic—sweating heavily.

"I'm hot, I'm so hot," he says, trying to rip his shirt off. "I need to get out of my clothes."

I don't know anything about his medical history, but he's pale and so thin he seems fragile. The look in his eyes tells me something is seriously wrong.

His wife, who is sitting next to him, says, "He hasn't been feeling good. He's been having some abdominal pain."

There's a high degree of autonomy for nurses in the emergency department. When the ED gets really busy, doctors can't be in every room.

Linda, my preceptor, says to me, "I'm going to show you how to start the sepsis workup."

I studied sepsis in nursing school. It's a systemic infection that affects the whole body.

One of our residents comes in, examines the patient, and says he's not too worried about the man's condition. After he leaves, I look at Linda. I can tell she doesn't share the doctor's attitude.

"We're going to pull up our protocol," she tells me.

Linda and I get the patient on the monitor, then she asks me to get IV access. He's really hard to stick, and as I struggle, I start freaking out. Linda helps me, then she goes to send the blood work to the lab.

Even though I have nothing left to do, I stay with the patient. I don't want to leave him.

When I look at his monitor, I see he's in asystole, which means he doesn't have a heartbeat. He's flatlining.

As if in slow motion, I look at him, this man who now doesn't have a pulse, then I look at his wife, then I'm on top of him, doing chest compressions on a patient for the first time, cracking his ribs—possibly even breaking them—and yelling as loud as I can, *"I need help in here!"*

A call for help in the ER brings everyone running. Linda has been gone for only a few minutes. She charges inside the room and says, "What the hell is going on? What happened?"

A nursing assistant takes over chest compressions. Nursing assistants are incredibly helpful that way; they tend to be the ones doing the chest compressions, allowing the nurses to take charge of medications, charting, the defibrillator.

I get off the man's chest and look at the whirlwind happening around me. I watch nurses set up for intubation and respiratory therapy and see the physicians who will perform the intubation.

The man's wife is crying. A nurse comes in, sweeps her up, and pulls her to the side. We don't believe in kicking family members out of the room during aggressive treatment (unless they don't want to be there) because it's hard for them to cope if they're alone and in the dark as to what's actually happening. It's better to have a designated person explain to the family members exactly what's going on and what we're doing to help their loved one.

I don't know what to do. I don't know where I fit in.

James, a male nurse I really look up to, says, "Come here,

Shannen. We're going to be on the defibrillator. I want to show you how to do it."

He explains what we're about to do next.

The most important actions in this situation are doing chest compressions and "bagging the patient," which means using a manual, handheld resuscitator to get air into the patient's lungs. CPR is briefly stopped every two minutes so we can see if the heart rhythm on the monitor is shockable.

James shows me how to charge the defibrillator and shock the patient. After two minutes of CPR, the nursing assistant stops compressions and we look at the monitor. The patient is in ventricular fibrillation. That's a shockable rhythm.

"Okay," James says to me, "it's go time."

The defibrillator is charged up. I look at the man and say, "Clear" as I hit the glowing red button on the defibrillator. The electrical charge causes his body to bounce a bit on the table.

Oh my God.

"You did it," James says. "Great job."

Chest compressions are immediately started again. After two minutes, we check and find he's got a pulse back. Shortly thereafter, he's transferred to the ICU.

I stand there reviewing everything that just happened while wondering if the patient is going to be okay—and that's the struggle nurses face when working in the emergency department. About 95 percent of the time we don't know if the patient is, in fact, okay after he leaves us because we never hear about that patient again. I know this, but I'm still struggling to cope with it.

During my debriefing with Linda, one of the new things

I learn is that the cracking sound I heard while doing chest compressions wasn't his ribs breaking. The sound is caused by cartilage cracking.

A week later, this man is still alive. I'm told he's alert and breathing. I ask Linda if I can go up and visit him. She says yes.

When I walk into his room, I see him sitting up in bed eating breakfast.

It's surreal. *Oh my God, we actually saved this man's life. And I helped. I did this.*

In that moment, I realize I'm an emergency room nurse.

"Do you remember me?" I ask him.

He studies me for a moment. "No," he says.

"I was one of the nurses who took care of you downstairs. I just wanted to see how you were doing."

He gets incredibly tearful. I sit with him and we cry a little bit as he thanks me. His only complaint is that his chest is still a little bit sore, which is understandable. Having this conversation solidifies in my mind that I'm doing the job I'm meant to do.

This experience of resuscitating someone and later being able to meet and talk with that person is, I learn, extremely rare.

It hasn't happened to me since.

DARLENE BURKE

Darlene Burke lives in Richboro, Pennsylvania. She started her nursing career working in a med-surg unit. For the past thirty-nine years she has worked at the same community hospital, where she is currently a nursing supervisor.

I'm in nursing school, working in labor and delivery and living in a dorm across the street from the hospital. The location is convenient because I'm following a mom who is ready to have a baby, and they call me when she's ready to deliver so I can be there for the birthing experience.

I arrive and go into the delivery room. Watching the mother give birth—it's all so very exciting.

I follow the baby boy to the nursery. My job is to wash him and the umbilical cord—or, more accurately, the umbilical stump, tissue that within one to two weeks will shrivel and fall off the baby's navel. Until that time, it's critical to keep the stump clean and dry.

I pick up a bottle of gentian violet, a bright purple solution with mild antibacterial properties. I squeeze too hard, and the solution spills across the baby's stomach and toes.

I watch it spread, panicking. As I'm trying to wipe up the solution and pat it dry, spreading the stain even more, the father knocks on the nursery window and says, "Let me see my baby."

I'm staring down in horror at the father's son. The newborn's belly—it looks like he has a port-wine stain, a birthmark caused by capillary malformation. I keep trying to clean the skin, but the stain isn't going away.

The father isn't going away either. He keeps knocking at the window, asking to see the baby.

I wrap up the newborn and hold up his son.

"Unwrap him," the father says. "I want to see him."

Reluctantly, my heart pounding in fear and tears beading in my eyes, I unwrap the child.

The newborn is completely discolored, to the point where he looks damaged.

The father's face goes white. "Oh . . . my . . . God."

I'm so devastated I start sobbing. I put the baby down and then go out to talk to the father. I apologize over and over again as I explain the accident I caused. He's great about it, even when I tell him it will take months for the stain to disappear, but I can't stop crying.

He leaves, then comes back with flowers to help calm me down. The passage of time has softened the moment. I can almost laugh about it now.

MARGARET CARMAN

Margaret Carman is the director of Emergency Nursing Advanced Practice at the Emergency Nurses Association. At University of North Carolina at Chapel Hill, she is a full-time associate professor at the school of nursing and practices in UNC's Department of Emergency Medicine.

I'm so excited.

Today, my son turns two. I can't wait to get home and celebrate his second birthday. It's 1990, and I've just started working as a nurse in an emergency department.

I'm coming off shift when the ER gets a call about an incoming patient—a pediatric cardiac arrest. It's a little girl, accompanied by her grandmother. I don't know it at the time, but she's suffered not one but two cardiac events.

The girl, I find out, somehow got hold of the grandmother's desipramine, which is an antidepressant. She climbed under a coffee table, ate the pills, and went into cardiac arrest.

And now the little girl is coding. She's not breathing, her heart isn't working, and we have an entire team—nurses and technicians, doctors and respiratory therapists—working on her and hoping against hope that we can bring her back.

We can't.

We finally call it.

The grandmother is devastated. She has no idea how her granddaughter got her hands on those pills.

The girl's mom is now on the way to the hospital to say goodbye to her daughter. There's no way I can make this right, but I can get this child ready for her mother to see her one last time, put a warm blanket on her.

The girl is lying on the table, wearing a pair of little red Mary Jane shoes. I'm cleaning her up when I notice she's wearing an ankle bracelet with a small medallion. I lean forward and see the girl's date of birth engraved on it.

She shares the same birthday as my son.

The moment is so upsetting and, at the same time, so profound. I go try to comfort the grandmother.

In my car, driving home—that's when I process things like what happened today. I don't fall apart, but I think about it. Was I able to perform one little thing that provided a small measure of comfort? Was I there for someone?

I believe that God made me to help people. I know that might sound corny, but nursing is my calling. I don't do a whole lot of good things—I don't build houses for Habitat for Humanity, I don't give hundreds of dollars to charity—but, by God, I'm there for people, usually at the end of their lives, when they need me.

When I arrive home, I hug my son, knowing I'm so lucky to have him.

PATRICK KAPPAUF

Patrick Kappauf was born and raised in Delaware and currently lives in its largest city, Wilmington, where he works as an ER/ trauma nurse at a level-one trauma center.

As a punk-rock kid living on the streets, trying to make it as a musician, I don't respect nursing as a profession in any way, shape, or form.

I have no reason to. I'm a drummer. Music is my life. My passion. My first love.

I join a rockabilly band out of Albuquerque, New Mexico. For the next few summers, I tour with these guys. The band doesn't make enough money for me to pay the bills so, during the winter months, I work at Starbucks.

I experience this weird kind of dichotomy. When I'm on tour, I'm playing in front of thousands of people; I sign autographs and do all sorts of cool stuff. Then I return home, and I'm standing behind the counter at Starbucks taking crap from people.

It's soul-sucking.

I start to look for another source of income. I'm thinking phlebotomist. I've used drugs—had a fairly long stint with drugs and alcohol before getting into recovery—so I have a history with needles. Maybe I can take my past and put it to some sort of good use.

A technical school near me offers certifications in phlebotomy and a career path to become a medical technician. It's been a long time since I've been in school. I sign up, thinking I'll barely scrape by in class to get the certifications I need, but when I start working with the instructors, I end up doing really, really well. The anatomy and physiology—everything sort of clicks. It all feels effortless. I'm able to speak the medical language, and I start working toward becoming a medical technician.

While in school, I get a job as a patient-care tech in the emergency department. It's part of a four-month internship. Two weeks in, I'm told the hospital wants to hire me when I graduate.

I end up liking what I do so much that I quit the band.

One day, I'm assigned to watch a woman who is here for a psych evaluation. She has a history of multiple personality disorder. She's also a professional kickboxer. My job is to sit with her and make sure she doesn't hurt herself or anyone else.

Everything's going fine. She's sitting in bed and I'm reading a book and keeping an eye on her when all of a sudden, she jumps up and runs away.

I chase after her, catch her from behind, and wrap my arms around the upper part of her chest to hold her. She bites down on my arm.

Locks her jaws in a death grip and won't let go.

She's biting down as hard as she can—the pain is excruciating. I'm getting ready to punch her when one of the nurses grabs my free arm. I can't punch a patient. If I do, I'll probably lose my job.

Doctors are all over us, trying to pry her jaws open, but she's really strong, and her mouth is clamped down hard on my arm. When they finally get her off me, security guards tackle her, drag her back to the room, and put her in four-point restraints.

My wound is pretty awful-looking and painful as hell. After it's cleaned, they give me a tetanus shot and some Tylenol, and the entire time I'm thinking, *This sucks. I can't believe this happened.*

But there's another thought, one that's been developing for quite some time. Working in the ER has given me a lot of respect for nurses. I've been watching what they're doing, the amount of autonomy they have, and it blows my mind. They're loudmouths and they cuss a lot and they have a really sick sense of humor, which you need to get through this job.

There's a lot of teamwork on a very level playing field. They speak to the janitor and the surgeon in equally respectful tones. *These nurses—these are my people. I could definitely do this. This totally makes sense to me.*

After graduation, I end up working full-time at the hospital while going to nursing school.

As a nurse, I watch people die every day.

The scrubs I wear act as a suit of armor. The physical barrier creates a clinical, matter-of-fact mindset. *I'm going to see whatever I'm going to see today. Whatever happens is going to happen. And when I see something bad, I won't dwell on it or get emotional about it because there's too much shit going on, and I have a job to do.*

I don't think a lot of people understand how many times during a shift a nurse is forced to switch gears. One day, I'm working on a three-year-old who was found floating in a pool. The child can't be resuscitated and dies. I'm mentally, physically, and spiritually wrecked when I walk back out to the triage hallway.

A guy with a sprained ankle lying on a gurney sees me and starts cussing me out because he's been in the hallway for an hour waiting for someone to take him back to a room.

I so badly want to tell him off, tell him what I've just witnessed. But I can't do that. I have to quickly shift gears.

I tell myself he doesn't know what I just walked away from, that it's my job to make sure he doesn't know. So while he's cussing me out, I take a few seconds and downshift. When he finishes his verbal onslaught, I say, "Yeah, I know. I'm really sorry you've been waiting for so long."

Nurses also deal with a lot of physical abuse. One day a gentleman comes in and tells the triage nurse that he's hearing voices ordering him to hurt other people and kill himself. Before the nurse can say or do anything, the man takes off inside the ER.

I'm walking down a hall, about to go into a room to check on a patient, when the man blasts by me, running full speed. A nurse is chasing after him.

"You have to stop him," she says to me. "He's running toward the outpatient part of the hospital."

There are a lot of people walking around that area. I run after him. Corner the guy near outpatient radiology.

He turns and punches me in the face.

I remind myself that I can't punch a patient and go into modified attack mode. I grab him by the waist. He manages to get an arm around my neck and starts choking me.

People are coming out of radiology, watching us in horror.

Just as I'm seeing stars and right before I'm about to pass out, I jam my thumb into his eye. He lets go and starts punching me in the face, and that's when security arrives and breaks us apart.

My face is busted up a little, and I have marks around my neck. As pictures are taken of my injuries to document the incident, I'm told the guy who just attacked me somehow escaped from the psych unit, which is typically locked down. After I'm cleaned up, I meet with management to tell them my side of the story. I don't get into trouble, but the hospital is very concerned about how this happened.

Once in a while, you get patients who appreciate what you do. I have a female patient who has been knitting for a good chunk of the day she's spent in an ER bed, and when I go check on her, she hands me a potholder.

"I didn't know what to make you," she says, "but you said you cooked, so I thought you might be able to use this."

"Thank you. That's very thoughtful." And I mean it.

I still have that potholder, and I do use it.

One of the best times I have in the ER involves a guy with chronic diarrhea.

And it's bad. Really, really bad. Just water pouring out of this guy's ass.

And it's an absolute nightmare getting him cleaned up, and he's taking up a lot of my time, to the point where I'm almost neglecting my other patients.

One of the ER nurse managers comes up to me and says, "Why don't you go ahead and put a rectal tube in the guy?"

Rectal tubes, I know, are often used to prevent soiling in critically ill patients. They send one over. I stare at it. *Never mind that I've never inserted one before,* I tell myself. *I've put plenty of tubes in patients, in nearly every possible hole.*

No one in the ER knows how to use this contraption. Four people come back with me to the patient's room. I'm standing behind the guy with my hand in his ass trying to figure out how to put this tube up there, and every once in a while, he shits all over the place.

At some point, the stress gets so great I can't help but laugh. It happens to all nurses. We can't help but see the humor in the ridiculous situations we find ourselves in.

BETHANY EDMONSON

Bethany Edmonson was born and raised in Texas. Since 2004, she has worked as an ER nurse in Dallas.

You have to completely undress some ER patients. They don't teach you that at nursing school. With trauma patients especially, it's important to have them completely undressed so you can evaluate them because you have no idea what you might find.

The homeless lady in the ER exam room is complaining of abdominal pain. As she undresses, she says, "Be careful, because I have my pet with me."

"Where's your pet?" I ask. "Is it in your bag? Is it a dog or a cat?"

"No, it's a bird."

"Where is it?"

"It's underneath my jacket."

I don't see a bird. But as she's getting undressed, it falls out of her jacket.

The bird is black and has a couple of blue feathers. It's wrapped in a little blanket. It's also clearly been dead for quite some time.

Okay, I tell myself, *she has a dead animal as her pet. It's her companion, so I guess we'll all have to go along with it.*

It's kind of gross but also kind of funny. When I leave the room, I can't help but break down in laughter.

Our homeless population also has a unique sense of humor. One lady who comes in frequently stops by one day and says, "I would like to present you with a picture of my mug shot."

I don't know how she got a copy of her mug shot or why she felt the need to bring it to us. "Thanks, Mrs. Brown. You made our day."

Some of the objects we pull out of people's private areas are pretty, pretty impressive. I've pulled out a sixteen-inch cucumber and a glass beer bottle. And the patients always say, "I have no idea how that got up there." They never want to tell us the full story.

Some days I ask myself, *What on earth just happened? Did I really pull a cucumber out of someone's bottom? Did I really just find a dead bird in a lady's jacket?*

JENNIFER

Jennifer lives in California and works as a nurse in a major hospital.

When you're an ER nurse, you don't have time to have feelings, let alone dwell on them. What emotions you do have, you have to isolate and control. Move on and keep going. If you can't do that, you won't make it as an ER nurse.

Today, I think I might not make it. I'm afraid.

Afraid that I won't be able to cut it. Afraid that I won't be able to do what needs to be done. Afraid that when something awful happens, I won't be able to keep going.

That something awful is already happening, and it's coronavirus. The reality of its deadly reach is just beginning to sink in.

Right before people die, they do what we call "guppy breathing," where they gulp air like a fish out of water. The woman who comes into the emergency department is breathing this way. She's dying.

From COVID.

The woman stares at us, tears running down her face, while we work to get her as comfortable as possible.

The moment is heartbreaking. And chaotic.

The doctors and the medical staff are talking openly about the fact that she is going to die. The woman can still hear us. She's aware.

And absolutely terrified. I can see it in her eyes.

What she's seeing right now are strangers dressed in gowns, gloves, masks, and face shields. We're all gowned up in protective gear that can't be removed while we're with a patient.

Most people don't realize that this whole COVID pandemic has caused a major shift in medical treatment. The human touch is almost gone.

I can't take off any of my gear, but I can hold this woman's hand.

"It's going to be okay," I say, wiping away her tears with a tissue. "I'm right here with you. I know this is scary, but I'm going to be right here with you."

It hurts my soul that this woman is going through this without her family. I've never shed a tear in front of a patient before, but this time I can't help myself.

The last thing this woman sees is my masked face.

I'm still gowned up and wearing my protective gear when I head downstairs to another treatment room. There the chaos repeats—another woman suffering from COVID is having problems breathing. Her oxygen saturation levels are down in the sixties, and she's getting combative because she's hypoxic. The organs in her body are starved for oxygen.

She's going to need to be intubated.

I start her IV. Once people bring me the preparatory medications, I get her on a monitor and administer them. The doctor intubates her. I put in an orogastric tube to decompress the stomach, get all the gases out.

When everything is done, I take a step back.

I may be scared, but I'm still here. I'm an ER nurse.

KAYLEIGH GIBSON

Kayleigh Gibson is a registered nurse in Cincinnati, Ohio. She currently works in the ICU.

Everyone who works in the ICU deals with patients who are so incredibly sick—and with families who are so incredibly scared.

I speak from experience—as a nurse, and as a patient.

As a toddler, I suffered from seizures. I spent a lot of time at Children's Hospital, where I was diagnosed with a brain tumor. Fortunately, the tumor was benign, but I had to undergo brain surgery.

I don't remember much about that time, but my mom and dad never forgot it. My mom always spoke about how terrified she and my dad were, how appreciative they were of the nurses—their calming presence, their dedication to making sure my parents understood everything that was going on with my care.

My mom talked about how the doctors came in and out, but the nurses were always there. They spent time with me, walked around the hospital with me, brought me balloons. Everything they did was special, and they made my parents feel like I was in really good hands.

Hearing these stories as I grew up had a profound impact. Nursing became my calling. I wanted to affect my patients' lives, make their toughest days better. And now I do.

When COVID hits, I'm new in the ICU. It's instantly clear there's emotion involved in working here, a lot more than there was in my previous job on a medical floor at another hospital.

I'm constantly riding a roller coaster of sad cases. COVID patients are separated from everyone, so they're facing not only illness but isolation. I try my best to help my patients set up FaceTime or Zoom meetings with their families, but people with COVID can take rapid turns for the worse, and there isn't always time.

My latest patient inside the COVID ICU is a middle-aged woman who, I can tell, is getting ready to pass. I know she has a daughter, but there are no visitors allowed.

The thought of this woman dying alone is unimaginable. I gown up quickly and go inside to be with her. As I sit and hold her hand, all I can think about is the woman's daughter. The fact that she isn't able to be here with her mom breaks my heart.

After the woman passes, I call her daughter. She's crying and I start to cry too. These situations, losing a patient, are so, so hard on me, and they never get easier. Every time it happens, it's equally awful.

My other COVID patient that day is a young mom who is thirty-four weeks pregnant. She's short of breath, which is normal for a woman at this stage of pregnancy, but because she has COVID, she's decompensating—getting worse—pretty quickly.

I get together with the medical staff, and we decide that it's best that she delivers her baby right now.

But this is the COVID ICU, not labor and delivery, so we have to improvise. We set up a room next door for the baby. We also have to deal with a dangerous, potentially life-threatening issue: When the baby is born, the woman will experience a fluid shift that will possibly cause her to go into some form of cardiac arrest. Ten medical people, some of them specialists from different departments within the hospital, stand outside the room, waiting to be summoned in the event of an emergency.

Nurses influence how patients and their families perceive what's happening around them. The woman's husband can't be here with his wife, but I can set up an iPad so he can watch the delivery at home.

The couple is so sweet and calm and appreciative.

A labor and delivery nurse, an ob-gyn, and I assist the woman with her delivery. We bring the baby to the other room and then I go back to work on stabilizing the mom.

She ends up doing well. I take care of her for a couple of days, and a week later, she's healthy enough to go home with her baby.

I don't know that I could have handled the situation as gracefully as the couple did.

But I try. I always try.

Helping patients and their families is not only a privilege—it's my reward.

DEVYN WELLS

Devyn Wells lives in northern California and works full-time in an emergency department.

I hate to judge people by their looks, but when someone tattoos his face, it makes me wonder about his mental status.

The young guy who walks into the emergency department has shaved off his eyebrows and replaced them with blue-inked spiderweb tattoos filled with some kind of writing. He's painfully thin, and he looks homeless.

"I'm just... I'm not well," he tells the nurse next to me at the triage desk.

"Physically or mentally?"

"Mentally. Definitely mentally." He sighs. His entire neck is tattooed. He's wearing mascara and has long hair that cascades over his shoulders. "I just want it all to, you know, end," he says. "The sooner the better."

"What's your name?"

He smiles. "Angel."

This guy is definitely not one of our "frequent fliers"—patients who are here a lot, usually homeless people who come in when it's cold or raining and say they're feeling suicidal so they can rest and eat a sandwich. I'd remember seeing a guy like this.

There's no question in my mind he's...off. Could be a drug-induced psychosis. Or he could be legitimately crazy.

I don't claim to be the best judge of psych patients but working in the ER has made me much more experienced. Not long ago, a young girl came in. She was what we call "gravely disabled"—her thought process was compromised, maybe because she'd fried her brain with drugs or maybe because she had a psychiatric condition that made her unable to formulate a real-world plan. Still, while she had some issues, she seemed functional.

That assessment changed when a hospital aide gave her a magazine. The girl removed the staples and proceeded to swallow them, thinking they would kill her. They didn't, but we had to X-ray her abdomen to make sure she would pass them in her stool.

We have a twenty-nine-bed ED. It's always busy, so we have potential psych patients wait on beds in the hall where the hospital staff can keep a close eye on them.

This is a recent policy change. We used to let them wait in the lobby until a young woman strung out on meth took out her pipe and lit up next to a pregnant woman. The meth-head thought her actions were perfectly reasonable, so she got really pissed at us when we asked her to leave, saying we were overreacting, and she created such a huge scene that security had to drag her kicking and screaming out of the hospital.

I take the guy to the hall bed, wondering if he's on meth. It's a huge problem here in northern California, and the drug often makes people suddenly turn violent. I'm five two and a hundred and thirty pounds. If this guy goes after me, I'm screwed. That said, I do have a surprisingly accurate left jab.

I'm working at the nurses' station when I receive word that a room with a bed has opened up. I go to retrieve Angel.

Before a psych evaluation, a patient has to be given a full medical exam. I escort Angel to the room, but I don't go in there with him. I ask him to put on paper scrubs, and while he undresses, I stand in the hall, the door cracked open in case I need to rush inside. We used to have psych patients change in the bathrooms. That stopped when a girl broke a bathroom light and tried to use the shards to cut herself.

As Angel is changing, one of the techs, a guy named Tony, comes rushing up to me. His face is pale as he leans forward and whispers in my ear: "That guy in there? We found a machete wedged between the mattress and bed frame."

My stomach drops.

"Security quietly confiscated it," Tony says. "I already called the police."

They arrive quickly. The way the cops speak to Angel gives me an inkling that this guy was involved in something bad.

But they don't arrest him. Angel is given a psych evaluation and sent to the psychiatric hospital.

While I don't know what the diagnosis is, the outcome makes sense, given that he came here with a *machete*.

A few days later, the news is buzzing all over the ED. A coworker of mine who is also a good friend comes over to me and says, "Did you hear about that guy Angel?"

"No. What's going on?"

"Remember that murder in San Francisco back in February—the body the police found stuffed in a suitcase in the bay?"

My thoughts are already running to Angel when my friend says, "Police ran the DNA on the machete. It's the one that guy Angel brought into the hospital. He confessed to the police. They also think he chopped up some other people in San Francisco and put them in boxes."

Going into work that day, I'd had no idea I would come into contact with a serial murderer. That's what makes this job exciting—when you walk through the door, you have no idea what your day is going to be like. No two days are ever the same.

JOHN ANTONELLI

John Antonelli served in the army for five years. He worked in EMS and law enforcement before becoming a nurse. He currently works as an ER nurse.

I get a call about a two-year-old boy who has been hit by a four-wheeler—an ATV—in a small, rural town. His father, the driver of the ATV, didn't see his son standing in front of him; he throttled down and ended up smacking the boy on the back of the head.

When I arrive with Roland, my EMS partner, we find a lot of blood. I assess the situation and discover that the boy has lost about an eighth of a cup of brain matter.

The trauma center is thirty miles away. We load the boy into the ambulance and immediately intubate him and start IVs. We drive as fast as we can.

Later, after we drop him off, I'm cleaning and packing the equipment away, and all I can think about is the kid's brain matter. Patients don't make it back from a critical loss like that. There's just no way.

I have the next five days off, but I can't stop thinking about this kid. It was by far the worst call in my EMS career.

What am I doing here? I keep asking myself. *I don't want any part of this. This is awful.*

EMS is based out of a local fire department. I'm in the bunk room with Roland when one of the volunteer fire-fighters comes in and says, "Hey, John, you're not going to believe this."

"Believe what? What's happening now?" All I feel is dread, wondering what I'm about to walk into next. Last week sucked, and whatever this guy is about to say is going to suck too.

"That kid you guys ran last week," the fireman says. "He's home."

What I'm hearing…it's not possible. There's no way that kid survived.

"He had a metal plate put in his head," the fireman says. "He's back home. He's playing. He has zero deficits."

It's a miracle. There's no other word to describe it.

This unexpected news opens up a floodgate of emotions. I end up sobbing in absolute joy. Roland does too.

Years later, when I'm working as a nurse in the ER, we get a seven-year-old who fell out of a treehouse. He comes into the hospital acting normal. He's sitting on the bed and suddenly he just falls backward, eyes rolling up into his head.

He goes into full cardiac arrest.

We work on him for fifty-four minutes.

He dies.

I come from the military and from law enforcement, and there's this stigma around showing emotion. You're supposed to push it down. You're the tough guy. You just deal with it as part of the job. But burying it deep down—that's not part of the job. You have to talk to someone, whether it be a priest, family member, friend, or counselor. If you don't—if you just keep it stored up—it's going to eat you alive. It's going to destroy not only your career but who you are as a person.

I'm in a leadership role now where I teach a lot of new nurses, and I constantly stress how important it is to feel your feelings. It's okay to be vulnerable. It's okay to hurt, to cry. It's okay to feel that loss. You can visit that place; you just can't live there.

I also share the outcomes of the two young boys I treated.

Sometimes, I tell them, you get to be a part of a miracle. Other times, no matter how well you do your job, it just doesn't work out. People are going to live, and people are going to die. You have no control. You just have to do your job.

TARA CUCCINELLI

Tara Cuccinelli grew up in Louisville, Kentucky. She studied nursing on an ROTC scholarship and served eight years in the military, deployed overseas, then worked for twenty-one years in the ER. Tara now works as a school nurse.

The little girl who's rushed into the ER looks like she's simply resting. She is probably two or three and has dark hair and big, brown eyes. There isn't any blood. All of her injuries are internal. She and her mother were just involved in a severe car accident.

The girl was in her car seat when the collision happened. Her chest appears bisected—pale from the nipple up and purple below the nipple. That clear line of demarcation makes me think she has an aortic dissection—a life-threatening condition where blood surges through tears in the inner layer of the aorta, the large blood vessel that branches off the heart's muscular pumping chamber.

Aortic dissection is, more often than not, fatal.

The mother is beside me, holding her daughter's hand and screaming hysterically as I perform CPR. I'm able to get blood flowing to the upper part of her chest, but not the lower part. I keep working, knowing it's futile but not wanting to stop.

"My baby," the mother screams over and over again. *"Not my baby."*

All of us in the room work on the girl longer than we normally would have, wanting her to live. She looks like she's just asleep, and a part of me believes she might wake up.

It doesn't happen.

I'm in tears. All the nurses in the room are crying. The doctor is crying. As I walk into the hallway, a door to another room opens. A red-faced patient glares at me and yells, "I need my pain medicine!"

Be thankful you can yell, I want to say. *Because the mom in that other room is never going to hear her daughter yell again.*

I wish people who came into the ER would understand that if we don't get to you right away, it means you're stable, that there's someone who is sicker than you. If you're waiting, that's a good thing. It's when we all rush in and jump on you that you should worry.

Although nurses are busy, we're doing the best we can—always trying to do more with less. Our hearts hurt for the people we can't get to right away and ache for the ones we can't save.

LIZ MARTINEZ

Liz Martinez worked as an ER nurse for fifteen years. She now works as a pre- and post-op nurse, helping patients prepare for and recover from outpatient surgeries.

There's a saying among nurses: "There's the right way of doing things, and then there's the real way of doing things."

Nursing school teaches you about disease processes and how to care for patients in the hospital. But I learn how to be a nurse from working alongside other nurses.

As Thanksgiving approaches, I confront another real nursing tradition: Nurses generally don't have weekends and holidays off. I'm a single mother, and it's the first time ever in my life I've been away from my family on a holiday. I'm feeling kind of sad for myself, but even though I'll miss gathering around the table with my family, I know they're there for me.

When you work in the ER, your patients leave you and you never know what happens to them. Did they live? Did they die? What was their outcome?

A woman at one of the casinos near our hospital goes into cardiac arrest in a bathroom. Someone performs CPR on her, and she's brought into the ED. We immediately hook her up to a monitor and get an ECG. The readings indicate she's having an ST-elevation myocardial infarction, or a STEMI. A STEMI is the most serious—and deadliest—heart attack, caused by a blockage in one of the major arteries supplying oxygen-rich blood to the heart.

After giving her medications and CPR, we get her back. Now we have to bring her to the cardiac cath lab at Harper Hospital. A resident physician, one of our transport techs, and I load the woman into the elevator.

As we're going down, her heart stops again.

I climb on top of her and do CPR in the elevator and all the way through the underground tunnel that connects the Detroit Medical Center to a collection of hospitals, including Harper. We manage to get her to the cath lab team.

Later on, I'm told the woman is alive and awake. I decide to visit her.

She's profoundly grateful. Her only complaint is that her chest hurts from the CPR. We broke some of her ribs.

Detroit is as rough as people say.

It's my first day as a tech at Detroit Receiving; I'm still in nursing school.

I'm working one early afternoon when we get a page. A young man has been in a motor vehicle accident. When he's brought into the trauma room, he goes into cardiac arrest.

We do CPR and get him resuscitated. He has a heartbeat again. He's intubated, so the ventilator can breathe for him.

He's stable. But when we move him down to the trauma module for monitoring, he crashes.

The charge nurse grabs me by the shoulders, stations me by the patient's bed, then hands me internal defibrillator paddles. "Hold these until you're asked for them," she tells me, "then press this button right here."

They perform a thoracotomy, which is where you cut open the patient's chest on the left side to gain rapid access to the heart. It's done only in a dire situation, the thoracotomy—it's a heroic medical Hail Mary.

We do everything we can to save this young man's life. He ends up passing away.

One night in 2011, while working the midnight shift, I take a cigarette break. I'm walking back in when a gentleman comes up to me holding a Dirty Harry revolver—one of those big ol' guns with the long, shiny barrels. He's bleeding profusely from his abdomen.

"I need your help, ma'am," he says. "I've been shot."

"Okay, I need you to put down the gun. We can't help you if you have a gun, I'm sorry."

I run inside and grab a wheelchair. Security—actual sworn police officers who work at the hospital—accompany me outside.

The man has put down the gun. Security retrieves it, and as I roll the man into the hospital, he says, "You all need to know, I have HIV, so everyone has to wear gloves."

What a lot of people don't realize about ER nurses is that we are always jumping out of one fire and into another. One moment you're standing next to a bed where a patient's chest is cracked open and you're doing everything you can to bring that person back to life, and then you literally turn around and take care of the next patient. There is no reprieve, no *Well, let me sit down and process what I just went through.*

There's no time to get adjusted to it. I don't think you ever really deal with what you see and do. Those mental scars remain for the rest of your life. I don't remember every patient who died, but I do remember many of them.

They stay with you even if you talk about it and get it off your chest. On really awful days, I'll go out with coworkers, have a glass of wine, and talk through things so when I go home to my family I can act as normal as possible.

Experiencing the worst day of someone's life every time you go to work changes the way you look at things. I do my best to hide what I've seen from the people in my life—and there's no doubt I have PTSD.

Absolutely awful incidents stay in my mind—like the mom and her three kids who were setting off fireworks at a car wash. The mom lit a mortar, and when nothing happened, she went over and looked down at the device. That's when the mortar went off. She lost the majority of her face.

Every Fourth of July when I see fireworks, I immediately think about her and what her poor children had to experience.

A lot of my profession involves pushing some things down so you can keep going. It wasn't until I started dating my husband, who is a firefighter, that I felt like I could talk about the things I see. Because of his job, he understands. He experiences the same things I do. Because he understands all my terminology, I don't need to alter my language to try to explain things to him.

It's an amazing relationship. Very therapeutic.

I'm down in Florida with my family and we're watching the local news when a story comes on about how a gentleman walked into a hospital through a standing metal detector and triggered an alarm. A police officer asked the man if he had anything in his pocket.

The man took out a grenade—and pulled the pin. The officers jumped on him and held his hand down so he couldn't let go of the safety lever and detonate the grenade. The hospital—the Detroit Medical Center—was evacuated.

"Yup, that's where I work," I tell my family. "That's my other home."

I leave the city to work at a suburban hospital. It's 2017 and I'm in the ER when we get a radio call: "We're bringing in an eleven-year-old with a self-inflicted gunshot wound."

The victim, I discover, is coming from the city where my stepkids go to school.

I begin to panic. Your worst fear as an ER nurse is that you're going to walk into a room and see someone you love.

My mind goes to the worst-case scenario. I text my husband: Where are the kids? Are they okay?

As I wait for him to answer, the eleven-year-old is brought in.

The victim is a boy. He's not one of my kids. I don't recognize him.

We get him stabilized and send him up to the OR. I've gotten to the point in my career where I avoid the operating room if I possibly can. I've seen enough horrible things to last me a lifetime, and today, I'm super-shook by what's happening.

I pass the family waiting area and see this strikingly beautiful woman sitting there, staring at nothing. I walk past the room, then decide to go back.

"Are you waiting for somebody?" I ask her.

"My son."

She's the young boy's mother.

She starts crying.

I sit with her. "They're working on him. They're doing every-thing they can," I say. "He's got some of the best doctors in there."

I keep speaking to her, trying to offer some degree of comfort. I ask if there's anyone I can call. She asks me to call her mom, who is at home watching her daughter, and her job. I call the woman's mother, and then I call the woman's place of employment to let them know she's at the hospital.

The young boy ends up passing away.

The mother kills herself several months later.

I have a family history of suicide. When someone ends his or her life, the family members and the other people left behind are saddled with so many unanswered questions. The mother's death hits me like a ton of bricks.

I keep thinking about the woman's daughter. The girl's brother is gone and now her mother is gone and she's all alone. I want that little girl to know when she grows up that she was on her mom's mind while she was sitting there waiting to learn about her brother. I don't want that girl to think, *Oh, my mom only cared about my brother and she couldn't get over the grief, so she ended her life.*

I decide to reach out to the aunt. I've never done anything like this before, and I don't know if it's inappropriate.

The aunt is really grateful that I've reached out. I don't know if it will bring any comfort to this little girl, but I need her to know about her mom. I need her to know.

VICTORIA LINDSAY

Victoria Lindsay grew up in Texas and joined the navy, where she was a gunner's mate. When she left the navy, she went to nursing school. She gravitated toward the ICU at first and then began working with heart-transplant patients. Victoria specializes in cardiothoracic-surgery nursing.

Certain patients are just dicks.

And I say that knowing that most of our patients are extremely sick.

I work mainly with heart-transplant patients and patients who are on a left ventricular assist device, or LVAD, which is a surgically implanted pump for those who have end-stage heart failure. The device isn't a forever fix, but it can buy the patient some time while he or she waits for a heart transplant.

A nurse is admitting a former patient of mine, a guy named Ben. He's standing next to his wife, and the nurse is explaining that Ben needs to drink this certain mixture before he heads down to get his CT scan.

"Nope," Ben says to the nurse. "I'm not drinking it."

The nurse is new, and she has no background with Ben.

I come in, look at him, and say, "You're going to drink this. It tastes like shit. You already know it."

Growing up in Texas, coming from a rough background and then working with weapons in the navy—I'm that asshole nurse who gets called a drill instructor because I don't put up with anyone's bullshit. "You're not lying in bed all day," I tell my patients. "You didn't come to the hospital to get surgery so you could lie in bed or sit on your ass, so get up."

My mom always told me I marched to the beat of my own drum. She also said, "Don't lie to people," which is why I don't have a filter.

Ben says he won't drink the mixture.

"You better start chugging," I tell him.

His wife bursts out laughing. She loves me because I'm so stern with her husband. And I have to be this way with him—very, very direct. Nurses in my line of work, we're type A personalities, very driven and rough around the edges.

I get floated regularly to ICUs. The ER at one hospital sends up a patient who is in severe pain. He tells me he's been constipated for a week.

Every person's bowel regimen is different. Some people go multiple times a day; some people don't go for days. Others go once a week. That's their normal, as they say.

"Do you go only once a week?" I ask. I have to ask about his history in this area because you don't want to make someone poop every day if he's not used to pooping every day.

"No," he replies. "I've been constipated for a week."

"What alternatives did you try?" The average person with minimal medical knowledge will drink some water or take a laxative or a stool softener. I've known people who will do an enema if they're a little freaky.

And then there's the thing that people don't like to talk about, called "disimpacting." If you come to the hospital severely constipated, someone will stick a finger up your butt, kind of give it a little whirl to try to get the poop out. The guy writhing in excruciating pain in front of me and my coworkers says he tried that, but he didn't use his finger.

"What did you use?" I ask.

"A butter knife."

It's been a long shift, and I need to make sure I heard him correctly. "I'm sorry, sir. Can you repeat that?"

"I shoved a butter knife up my ass."

Which, I soon discover, is why he's in such excruciating pain. When he shoved the butter knife up his rectum, he perforated it—meaning, in layman's terms, he ripped a little section up there in his butthole.

It's really hard to stay professional when you're told something like this. I've got a very unprofessional smirk on my face when I say, "Why didn't you try a spoon? You know, *scoop* it out?"

I'm getting these looks from my coworkers signaling *Get out of the room* because it's hilarious, and we're all trying not to laugh.

After a heart transplant, a patient doesn't necessarily leave the OR with the chest closed. There's a lot of trauma that happens—a lot of swelling and inflammation, a lot of fluid overload. Sometimes we have to take a patient with an open chest into the critical-care unit and get him or her stabilized. The chest can stay open for days until the inflammation goes down.

I try not to get attached to my patients. When they come to me, they're in bad shape. This is going to sound very dark, but the sooner people accept that death is a part of life, the sooner they can just move on with certain stuff.

Today, Ken, one of my former LVAD patients, is getting a new heart.

He smiles when he sees me. "You are the good-luck charm I was looking for today," he says.

"Why's that?"

"You prepped me for my LVAD. Your name is Victoria." He tells me he's from a town in a different country called Victoria. "And now you're prepping me for my heart transplant."

He gets all emotional and teary-eyed as I prep him for surgery.

"Just change your lifestyle," I tell Ken. "Whatever you were doing before, you need to really come at it from different points and change. You need to be able to eat healthy and exercise to the best of your ability."

Ken nods in agreement, but he doesn't know what I do.

Not everyone who gets a new heart actually takes care of it. I've seen heart transplants ruined pretty quickly over a few years because patients didn't control their diabetes. They end up basically throwing the whole damn heart away.

I've had heart-transplant patients come back in and say, "You know what? I'm just not going to take my immuno-suppression medication anymore."

And I say, "You do realize someone *died* for you, right? That this heart you've got could have gone to someone a little bit healthier or younger—someone who could have done something more with their life. But it was given to you, and now you don't want to take your fucking drugs?"

I believe in Ken.

"You have to go into this operation with a very positive mindset," I tell him, because I really do believe that if you think you're going to die on the table, you might. "You're going to do good. You're going to come out. And you're going to be given that second chance."

Nursing school doesn't prep you for real-world dealings with patients' families. A lot of them act like they know more than you do, or they overreact. I understand that they've been waiting for hours to see their loved ones, but sometimes when patients come out, they're bleeding a lot from their chest tubes, and you have to get them stabilized.

You want to tell the family: *Let us stabilize your loved one before you come back here and see blood all over the sheets and us doing chest compressions because we're trying to save him.* Family members see stuff like that, they tend to either pass out or freak out.

Of course, if I put myself in the family's shoes, I realize that if that were my mom or another family member—even my dog—I would not be in a good place either.

I have to accept the fact that everyone at the hospital does everything they possibly can, but sometimes a patient just doesn't make it. I don't like my emotions to get the best of me. I try to be very aware of that. When I have an awful day, I'll sit in my truck. *Okay*, I'll tell myself. *Your patient died.*

You had a rapport with him. You just have to give yourself a little bit of time.

I try hard not to take the bad stuff home with me. I run a lot to clear my mind. I like to go shooting and spend time with my two pit bulls, Jigsaw and Tank. It makes me realize that we need to really cherish the people who are in our lives and be grateful that they're still around.

ANDREW FESTA

Andrew Festa works in sales for a company that creates nurse-scheduling software and also works part-time as an ER nurse at a level-one trauma center in Long Island, New York.

I'm in Boston on the morning of September 11, 2001, when I get a call to come into work at St. Vincent's Hospital in downtown Manhattan. I've been a paramedic there for the past ten years.

All the bridges and tunnels into and out of Manhattan are closed, so the only way to get to the city is by boat or train. I drive my rental car to Bridgeport, Connecticut, and then take the next ferry out to Long Island, where I live. I arrive in the evening. I know I'm going to be at the hospital for a few days, so I grab as many clothes as I can before I jump on a train into the city.

When I arrive at St. Vinnie's, I learn patients will be assigned to hospitals according to their injuries. St. Vinnie's is the trauma center that's closest to Ground Zero, so all of the trauma cases will go to us. If someone is suffering from smoke inhalation or what have you, we'll bring them to either Beth Israel or New York–Presbyterian.

I get assigned a partner and hop in an ambulance. Everything south of Fourteenth Street is closed down, so there isn't any traffic. As we drive, I see cars and fire trucks abandoned on the side of the road.

Before coming to St. Vinnie's, I worked as a paramedic in Queens and saw a lot of awful things in a lot of awful places. Today I have this weird, eerie feeling, and it's heightened by the simple act of breathing. There's a burning sensation in the air and a smell that I can only describe as a mixture of death and dying.

I work for the next three days, and there's rarely a quiet moment. Then I'm alone with the sights and the smells that are all I can think about, that I'm still processing into dark memories. I know they'll stay with me forever.

Back in Queens, I developed a coping mindset. Anytime I started to feel bad for myself, I'd remember a patient who'd endured the unthinkable, like a dad who lost his wife and son on the same day. So however bad I'm feeling about whatever's going on in my life, I know from my experiences as a paramedic—like this awful, tragic event I've been working for the past three days—that there's always someone out there who has it way worse than me.

The idea of going to nursing school comes to me again.

I start to dismiss it the way I always do. *The problem is, I'm not a kid anymore. My life is different now. More complicated. I have a wife, children, and a mortgage.*

An ER nurse who has heard me talking myself out of going after my dream before says to me, again, "The time is going to pass no matter what you do. Just get your ass to nursing school."

This time, I listen to her. I'll go to nursing school.

I'm thirty-five years old.

The number-one rule about working in the ER is have zero expectations. Whatever you *don't* expect—that's exactly what's going to happen.

My time as a city medic has helped me prepare for the controlled chaos of the ER. As a medic, I dealt with incredibly uncontrolled environments. I'd have to treat patients in housing projects with no lights. I'd deal with someone in cardiac arrest knowing that people in the immediate area were carrying guns. Sometimes I would enter rooms where weapons were in plain sight.

In the ER, I'm never in that kind of danger, and I never have to work alone. I have the equipment I need and am part of a team of an attending physician and about ten other highly focused people.

During my time in Queens and working in Manhattan in the aftermath of 9/11, I learned that my job is to do my job. Focus on the airway. Focus on intubating or focus on making a wound stop bleeding. I'm not focused on the person. I'm focused on the task at hand.

Compared to my prior experiences, working in the emergency department is easy.

Then COVID strikes.

We all saw it coming back in early February, but I don't

think any hospital fully ramped up because we looked back at SARS-1, and that virus drifted away really quickly. The collective thinking was *Why should COVID be any different?*

Every hospital I know was completely unprepared.

In the beginning of April, it's early days of COVID. I wear the same N95 mask for two shifts. We have to ration PPE and reuse it. No one knows how contagious the virus is or if PPE is effective. There are just so many unknowns.

I see things in the ER I've never seen before.

A patient's clinical presentation does not always match the vital signs. Patients are profoundly hypoxic—suffering from oxygen deficiency—but they're not gasping for air. Their pulse-oximetry levels will be down in the seventies and sixties, which is where, theoretically, they should be going into respiratory failure, but they're not. They have a cough and a fever, but they're talking in complete sentences.

Then, forty-eight hours later, they crash and die.

In one ten-day span, all our COVID patients—most of them poor, obese, suffering from comorbidities, or all of the above—end up dying.

We've put sixty patients on ventilators. Each and every one of them died. I have two patients who are about to go on ventilators. "How long do you think I'll be on it?" each of them asks.

These two patients know they're facing long odds against survival, but I want to give them hope. Sometimes hope is all we have. "Every case is different, so it's difficult to say."

They both die.

I have another COVID patient, a guy who is probably around fifty years old. He has a few comorbidities, he's working hard to breathe, and he's getting really, really tired. He needs to go on a ventilator, but there isn't one available yet.

"I want to talk to my wife," he says, panting, drawing out each word.

"Sir," I say, calmly and gently, "I'm sorry, but we can't have any visitors—"

"She's in the waiting room. I want to talk to her. On the phone."

There really isn't any cell service in the trauma room, so he can't call or FaceTime her. He's not doing well. I know, deep down, that this might be the last time he'll be able to talk to his wife, so I give him the hospital's landline phone.

The conversation with his wife is very matter-of-fact. I get word that a ventilator has become available. I tell him, and he tells his wife. Then he looks at me and says, "She wants to know how long I'll be on it."

I don't see him having a different outcome than the other sixty patients. But he doesn't know this, and his wife doesn't know this, and I'm not going to be the one to tell either of them.

I want to give them hope.

"Every case is different, so it's difficult to say."

We put him on the vent. He dies later that evening.

Sometimes hope is all we have.

CORRIE HALAS

Corrie Halas grew up in Jackson, Tennessee; after graduating from nursing school, she moved to Utah and then to Colorado. Corrie is now a nurse consultant for workforce management and labor strategies.

At the hospital in Vail where I work, we see a lot of businesspeople and celebrities, especially in the orthopedic unit, renowned for its sports medicine program.

Affluent patients are not the easiest.

A Vegas hotel magnate under my care in the ER obsessively complains to me about the big air-conditioning units on the side of the building.

"I can hear the fans," he tells me yet again. "Those AC units should be on the roof."

I deliver the same consistent reply: "Sir, I didn't build the hospital. I have no control over that."

"Those fans are incredibly noisy."

Oh, come on, I want to say. *I've got better things to do than listen to you complain about AC fans. I've got some really sick people here, and you're not one of them.*

We get a lot of soccer players from the Middle East. They snap their fingers and demand food from outside the hospital—and then they order us to go pick it up. I'm young and sassy and a relatively new nurse, so I'll snap back, "You know, that's not going to work for me."

There are many wonderful patients. Six-year-old twin girls who recently got their tonsils out send me the cutest note, full of misspellings, inviting me over for dinner. If I have a boyfriend, the note said, I can bring him to dinner too.

I get a patient from Miami who was in a messy skiing accident. His name is Howie, and he needs a lot of help. His wife is with him the entire time he's there, helping him and helping us. He's funny as all get-out, and nice.

When it's time for Howie to leave, the physical therapist and I help get him into the limousine that will take him to Denver. Howie is so incredibly thankful for everything we've done for him that he starts throwing money out the window—twenties and hundreds.

"Howie," I say, "we can't take your money."

We pick it up and try to give it back to him, but Howie refuses to accept it. He throws more money out the window. The physical therapist and I quickly scoop up the bills and give them to the limo driver, and I keep saying, "Howie, we *can't* take your money."

When the limo leaves, people in the parking lot come up to us and ask, "Why is that man throwing wads of cash out the window? What's wrong with him?"

* * *

A male alcoholic patient going through the DTs starts throwing punches at us. I want to hit him back and then tie him down.

He escapes from the hospital—still wearing his gown. We're worried he might hurt himself, so a couple of us follow him through the streets of Vail, careful to remain out of reach of his fists. We call the police, say that one of our patients is loose. That he's kind of incoherent.

He walks into a hotel restaurant, sits down, and orders breakfast. A police officer comes in and goes up to his table.

"Hey, bro," our patient says. "What's happening?"

The cop sits down, and the patient starts talking like he's catching up with one of his buddies. Eventually, the cop manages to convince the patient to walk back to the hospital.

The brains of mentally ill people, I realize, sometimes just snap. My logic won't make any sense to them. It's up to me to figure out what mental state they're in and then try to find a way to communicate with them.

It's a subtle art, wasted on the young. Over time, I've honed my skills.

When I said to the Vegas hotel magnate, "I have no control over that," my words had an edge to them.

Now that I've lived long enough to know that there's no such thing as control, I'm telling the honest truth.

JODY SMITHERMAN

Jody Smitherman was born and raised in Boonville, North Carolina, and served in the navy. He's a trauma nurse in the emergency department and currently serves in a managerial role at a local hospital in Winston-Salem.

An older guy comes in dressed in workout clothing and sneakers. I'd say he's entering his golden years except that he looks so gray that I rush over and put him in a wheelchair.

"It's my back," he tells me as I take him into the ER. "Man, it hurts."

"I'm not trying to be rude, but you're as gray as a battleship, and you're sweaty."

"I'm sweating because I was working out."

"Humor me for a second, okay? I'm going to throw these electrodes—these round stickers right here—on your chest." I hook him up to the heart monitor and look at the screen.

He's having a massive heart attack.

Our hospital doesn't have a cath lab, but there's one in a facility that's ten minutes down the road. We transfer him there.

Later, I find out that he coded two minutes before arriving at the cath lab.

The survival rate for patients who code goes up dramatically if people immediately perform certain interventions. Because everything is ready as the guy is rolled into the cath lab, the team members put the shock pads on him and start compressions immediately.

Three months later, a man I've never seen before comes into the ER and gives me a big hug. "You saved my life," he says, his voice cracking, tearful.

"I think you have the wrong—"

"No, it was you. It was definitely you."

Maybe he's right. I'm hard to miss—I'm six feet tall, broad in the shoulders, and bald-headed with earrings, and I talk rather country. I'm also one of the two male nurses working here.

He then proceeds to tell me who he is—the guy who came in from the gym suffering from back pain. The one who looked like shit, I realize, and the one I'd seen for only twenty minutes before we shipped him down the road. Now I recognize him. He's so grateful and thankful that he's upright and walking.

It's happy outcomes like these that make what I do worth it.

PART TWO:

Night Shift

KELLIE TRAVERS

For the past twenty-three years, Kellie Travers has worked as a critical-care and ER nurse. She currently works in Palm Beach County, Florida.

The ER is never busy on Thanksgiving or Christmas, but the day after a big holiday is the worst because everyone is paying the price for overindulging. People who aren't supposed to have too much salt for medical reasons decide to partake and put themselves in congestive heart failure. Dialysis patients who know they aren't supposed to eat this or drink that decide to ignore their doctors' orders and then they come into the ER barely breathing.

And if it's a full moon? We're flooded with crazy people and women in labor.

If you think that's a myth, go work in the ER.

Amy, one of my ER nurses, comes up to me in the hallway and says, "I've got a bad feeling about one of my patients."

"Which one?" I ask.

She points to a man lying on a stretcher. He's conscious but his skin is a dusky-gray color.

"He came in complaining of severe abdominal pain," Amy says. "Dr. Smith has seen him. He's ordered the routine tests—blood work, urine, et cetera—but I think he may be suffering from an aortic dissection."

In a dissection of the aorta, the largest blood vessel in the human body, one or more layers of the vessel's wall ruptures, causing life-threatening internal bleeding. The aorta runs from the heart through the chest and down to the abdomen, and pain can radiate into the back. An aortic dissection requires emergency surgery—the sooner the better.

"Dr. Smith disagrees with me," Amy says. "Still, I'd like to put my patient in a room and get a monitor on him."

Amy is a great nurse, quick and keen. If she's got a bad feeling, it's probably valid.

"Put him in room six," I say, rushing off. "I'll speak to Dr. Smith."

I'm the charge nurse. Part of my job is administrative—managing shifts, creating schedules, overseeing patient admissions and discharges. I also do the work of a regular nurse. My main role is ensuring quality patient care, which sometimes means running interference between the doctors and nurses.

I find Dr. Smith at the docs' station, putting in lab orders.

"That male patient in the hall, the one suffering from abdominal pain," I say. "The nurse really feels this guy may have a dissection. We should do a CTA."

Computed tomography angiography (CTA) is a technique

involving an injectable dye and a CT scan; it allows radiologists to see if there are blockages or aneurysms in the chest and abdomen. The scan can also be used to determine if the patient has blood clots in his lungs.

"Can you please order a CTA?"

"Okay, fine," Dr. Smith huffs. "Whatever."

Sure enough, the patient has a dissection. He needs surgery. Now.

I call for an anesthesiologist, a cardiologist, and a surgeon. I need everyone in the OR in twenty minutes or there's a good chance this man will die.

The patient survives the operation. And it's all because Amy had a gut feeling.

"You owe that nurse an apology," I tell Dr. Smith. "She saved that guy's life."

Dr. Smith apologizes right away.

I don't think patients know what ER nurses actually do for them. That we're their advocates.

ER doctors sometimes see twenty-six patients at a time. They can be in a hurry, and their focus can be divided.

An ER nurse usually has only five patients. And nurses are fairly smart. We're going to look out for you. We're your eyes and ears to make sure you get what you need.

The people here in Florida can't drive in the rain. When I wake up and see that it's raining, I know the ER will be busy because there's going to be a million car accidents. Today is going to be even crazier because we're supposed to get hit by a hurricane, and I'm on the hurricane team.

It's like getting ready for a camping trip. I have to pack my own bag and bring my own food and an air mattress because I can't come home after my shift ends. I wave goodbye to my family and say a prayer, and during the drive to the hospital, I try to psych myself up so I'm ready when I walk through the door.

In the middle of the storm, we get people who are having heart attacks.

One is an older gentleman who recently had heart surgery. He's confused, and when I stand him up to help him walk, wrapping my arm around his waist, he coughs and spits a loogie on my shoulder. Then he literally pees and poops on my feet at the same time.

Well, that's a triple threat.

The roof on the hospital's second floor starts leaking because of the heavy rain.

The storm brings in a strange—and very disturbing—patient, a sixteen-year-old girl who comes into the ER with her boyfriend. Her face and mouth are swollen.

"She can't talk," the boyfriend says. "She, uh, shot herself in the mouth."

My job isn't to ask questions. That's the police's job, and the station is two minutes from the hospital. I tell the secretary to call them, and then I look at the boyfriend and say, "Sit down right there and wait for the police."

I call security to make sure the boyfriend doesn't leave. Then I grab an ER doc and half my team.

I can see the bullet wedged inside the top part of her mouth. It's small, probably a .22, and it looks like her hard palate prevented it from going through her brain. She's breathing okay, neurologically fine, but that doesn't mean this isn't a life-threatening situation. There could be swelling around her brain.

The girl can't talk, so I hand her my pen and say, "Write down your name and your mom and dad's phone number right here on the bedsheet."

The girl is very anxious. As she writes down the information, I call 911 and request emergency transport. The girl will need a trauma surgeon, which we don't have here, so she needs to be taken to St. Mary's Hospital.

A doctor generally handles calling the parents, but since the ER doc is on the other line with a trauma surgeon at St. Mary's, I have to make the call.

I get the girl's mother on the phone. I introduce myself quickly and then say, "Can you please tell me where you are right now?"

"I'm driving. Why? What's going on?"

I speak in a calm and measured tone. "I know you're driving, so please pull off the road for a moment, but *do not* panic." I wait while she stops the car. "Your daughter has been in an accident. She's—"

"*Accident?* Oh my God, what—"

"I need you to listen to me, and I need you to stay calm. I'm looking at your daughter right now, and she's alert. Her vital signs are stable, and she's completely neurologically intact. She has a bullet wedged in the top of her mouth."

The mother is freaking out. She starts asking questions about how it happened, but I don't have any answers for her. "We're transferring her right now for surgery. You need to go to St. Mary's."

I don't know how or why the girl shot herself. Or maybe

the boyfriend did it; I'll never know. That's the problem with working in the ER.

Later that day, I'm eating lunch with some of my coworkers. Another nurse, Amanda, walks in, looks at our colleague Bob, and says, "What's that on your shirt? Is that chocolate?"

Bob looks down at a small, dark blob. Amanda puts her finger in it, smells it.

"Nope," she says, "that's poop."

Bob was sitting there eating lunch and didn't even know he had shit on him.

A man who is suffering from chest pains comes into the ER with his two bodyguards. I recognize him right away because he's rich and famous. A lot of very wealthy people live on Palm Beach Island, and some come into the ER with bodyguards.

I put the man in a room with a drunk prostitute.

He's not happy. "I need you to remove that woman," the man says to me.

"I'm sorry, but it doesn't work that way. This is an ER. I know you're rich and famous and want privacy, but we don't have tons of empty rooms."

My shift ends, but the storm is still raging. I play Cards Against Humanity with some of the staff. I've never played it before. It's a really raunchy party game, and we have so much fun. It helps everyone relax so we can get through the storm and the chaos.

An unused part of the ambulatory area has been designated as our sleeping quarters. When I arrive, I see ceiling tiles scattered across the floor and water everywhere. All our stuff is soaked. The leak in the roof collected on the tiles until they fell from the ceiling.

I find a place to put my air mattress and lie awake, thinking about how nursing has made me grow into the person I am today. It's made me a good mother, because I see bad mothers. It's made me believe in angels, because I've seen miracles. It's definitely made me a stronger person and a better coworker. I work with these people for hours and days. They're my friends and my extended family.

I go off to do my rounds. Part of my job is to check the crash carts—the wheeled mobile units that contain all the medications, supplies, and devices that are needed in a code.

I knock on a door and enter the room. "Good morning," I say to the patient—an older woman who had some complications from a recent surgery. "Sorry to bother you. I'm just doing my routine check on your crash cart."

She looks at me and says, "You don't remember me, do you?"

I can't place her face.

"We met two years ago here in the ER," she says. "I came in with my husband. He'd just had open-heart surgery. He was going south, and then he started to crash. You came in and took over, told this person to do this, this person to do that, and not once did you lose your cool. My husband wouldn't be alive today if you hadn't walked in when you did and did what you did. You saved his life. I'll never forget your face for as long as I live."

I may have forgotten her face, but I'll never forget her words. These are the moments you live for as a nurse. These are truly the moments you remember the most.

MATT BENTLEY

Matt Bentley had a series of jobs before deciding, in his early forties, to go to nursing school. For ten years, he worked in the ER. Matt now works in nursing education.

I'm working the night shift with my friend Sarah when, at two a.m., the desk clerk comes back and says, "This young guy just showed up. He says he has an ingrown hair in his neck."

I look to Sarah. She's thinking the exact same thing I am: *Why would someone seek emergency treatment for an ingrown hair at two in the morning?*

We go to the waiting room. The patient's name is Barry, and his dad is with him. Barry's father accompanies us as we take his son back. We're a pretty small facility—a six-bed ER. The room I take Barry into is three gurneys with curtain partitions.

Sarah takes Barry's vital signs while I ask what I call

the annoying nurse questions—allergies, medical history, et cetera.

"He's been picking at this hair for the last week to ten days," the father says. "It's still there, and I think it might be infected."

Barry has a knuckle bandage covering his throat. I take it off and see a half-dollar-size opening in his soft tissue. I can see his trachea.

Sarah and I exchange *Oh, shit* looks.

"There's still a hair in there," Barry says. "If you look, you can see it."

The skin is all gray, necrotic-looking, and jagged.

"How did you do this?" I ask. "Were you just scratching it?"

"I used an X-Acto knife."

I can't believe what I'm seeing and hearing. It's amazing this guy didn't nick his jugular or puncture his trachea. I call the doctor, who is finishing up his fellowship in wilderness medicine, and ask him to come down and look at this real quick.

"There's still a hair in there," Barry tells the doctor.

"We're way past hair. You need emergency surgery."

The ear, nose, and throat doctor who's on call comes in, and he's gruff and cranky because it's three thirty in the morning. He looks at the wound and lays into the guy. "Why did you cut into your neck? Do you have any idea how serious this is? You know you could have died?"

I keep staring at the gaping wound. I don't know how the doctor is going to sew this back together.

COLLEEN CHAMPINE

Colleen Champine grew up in Mt. Clemens, Michigan. She has been in the nursing profession for twenty-six years and currently works as a registered nurse at a level-one trauma center.

When it comes to working in the ER," Andy says to me, "you either sink or swim."

Andy is an experienced nurse who takes brand-new baby nurses like me and teaches them the fundamentals of a hospital's emergency department—in this case, the ED at Detroit Receiving, Michigan's first level-one trauma center. Detroit can be a volatile city, and it takes special people to work at Receiving. This place isn't for everybody.

I've always wanted to work here. I'm an action junkie.

We're standing outside the hospital in front of the ambulance bay having a cup of coffee. This semicircular area where all the ambulances and emergency vehicles park is sectioned off from the main public entrance. A lot of nurses, medics, cops, and firefighters hang out here to talk. Take a break and decompress.

"You're going to be a good nurse," Andy says to me. "We've just got to fine-tune you a bit. We're going to—"

A car screams up the street and comes to a screeching halt right in front of us. Six guys jump out of the car. There's a guy lying in the backseat in a pool of blood.

Andy and I grab a stretcher. The man in the back has multiple gunshot wounds. We carry him to the code room, the place where we take patients who are on the edge of dying. The code room is staffed by an ER doc, people from X-ray, nurses, and a surgical trauma team.

We get his vital signs, put IVs in him, give him two units of blood, and send him off to the OR in just nine minutes.

At midnight, a motorcycle drives through the lobby's double doors and crashes into the entrance of the ER. The driver falls to the floor, bleeding. The motorcycle lies on its side, its motor still running, the wheels still spinning.

What the hell is this?

"I got shot on the freeway," the driver tells me over the roar of the bike's engine. "I knew if I got here to Receiving, I'd be okay."

We pick him up, put him on a stretcher, and take him into the code room.

The motorcycle is still running when I return. I don't know anything about bikes, so I grab a cop who is on his way out and say, "Do you ride?"

"Yeah."

"Can you pick up that bike and shut it off?"

He does. I sit with the bike next to me all night until the cops come get it.

*   *   *

The hospital has a module that takes the ER overflow during its busiest times. Tonight, we're short-staffed. I'm the only nurse, and I'm working with Dr. Ethan Anderson. He's about five feet tall and has a slight edge to him. Not everyone likes working with him, but I love Ethan's sarcastic and very dry sense of humor.

Our first patient thinks he's a werewolf. He's clearly psychotic and on some kind of drugs, and he keeps sitting up or kneeling on his bed and howling at the moon. Our next patient is a little old grandma who keeps calling Ethan an elf. The woman is terrified of elves, so she cries. Our third patient is a man who says he's giving birth.

"Oh my God, what is this?" I say to Ethan. "A full moon?"

I give a gown to the guy who says he's giving birth and say, "Get undressed."

Wolfman is howling in the corner and Grandma is trying to get off the bed, calling us fuckers, saying that we should have been aborted before we were born. Ethan and I can't help but laugh. We strap down Grandma so she doesn't hurt herself. Wolfman climbs up on her bed and howls.

"It's your fault I'm in here," I tell Ethan. "I picked overtime because you were working tonight. When we're out of here, you're buying."

"Yes, I am."

The guy who thinks he's giving birth has put on his gown. The fabric over his abdomen is covered in blood.

"Why is there blood on your belly?" I ask.

"Because I'm giving birth," the man replies. "To my baby."

"Number one, that's the wrong area. Number two, I know you have a penis, because I can see it. So what's the problem here?"

He lifts up his gown.

The man has a slice from his belly button almost to his nipple. What's even more disturbing—what my gaze is pinned on—is a round clump of hair sticking out from the wound.

I jump back about two feet and yell for Ethan over the Wolfman's howling and Grandma's curses.

"What is it?" Ethan yells back. "What's wrong?"

"Get over here. And grab the forceps."

He comes back with the forceps and stares at the clump of hair. It's several inches long and looks like a miniature horse's tail, and we're both trying to figure out what in the hell it is, what's going on here.

"You need to pull that out," I tell him.

"I'm not pulling that out."

"You're the physician. You're going to pull this damn thing out."

Ethan clamps down on the hair and slowly pulls.

Oh my Lord.

The hair is attached to a Barbie head.

This crazy man has "impregnated" himself with a Barbie doll.

Some of the man's intestines spill out. Now we've got to get him to surgery.

All of this is happening during the first half hour of work.

As a nurse, I do the best I can with each patient and then I move on because somebody else needs me. I learned that from my father, who was a cop. He taught me to do the best job I could with someone and then hope that the next person did the same.

That's my defense mechanism—do the best job I can and move on. I can't take this stuff home with me every night. In the emergency room, where so much trauma happens, reactions need to be a little callous. Feel sympathy, but don't feel empathy.

We get a very bad trauma, a woman who is five months pregnant. She was in the car with her boyfriend; he ran a stop sign, and a truck hit the passenger side. She's suffered extensive injuries—multiple lacerations to her liver and spleen, a fractured pelvis, and a collapsed lung. She's unresponsive and not breathing well.

We intubate her. We put in chest tubes, crack open her chest, and start cardiac massage.

She and the baby die.

We're all looking at each other in a state of shock. A couple of our regular drunks come in. Usually they're singing, and normally, we're like, *Okay, whatever,* and we sing a little bit with them.

Tonight, they're not singing. Even they can tell that something is very wrong.

There's a reason why cops and nurses get together. We deal with the same types of situations and people.

I've been a single mother since I was a nursing student, and "Mama" is what everyone calls me. Randy, an officer and dog handler with the state police, is much younger, but we instantly became friends. He has a genuine love of people and wants to do the best he can for the community. There's a thirty-year age gap between us, and while I'm a bit jaded and have a somewhat hard exterior—I've been a nurse for twenty-six years, seen the best and worst in people—when Randy's around, I'm reminded of why we do what we do.

He's a remarkable human being. Randy and his girlfriend are into dog rescue. They foster and train dogs, some of which have potential to work for the state police. Most go to good homes.

I work a set schedule: Sunday, Monday, Tuesday. Anytime Randy comes into the ER, he seeks me out and makes the same request: "I want you to see this new dog I got. Come outside and look at him and give him a dog treat. Then I want a hug from you."

This has been going on for years. Randy always insists that I see his dog. It forces me to take a break from the craziness of the ER.

It's the Tuesday before Thanksgiving, and the ER is on fire, metaphorically—trauma code after trauma code and medical code after medical code. I'm working triage when Randy comes in and brings me a cup of coffee. He tells me how much he loves me.

"Yeah, yeah, I know," I say, laughing. "Now get out of here, I'm too busy for you today."

He kisses the top of my head like I'm his mother and walks out the door.

That night at 6:15, an hour before my shift ends, I'm standing at my desk with two Detroit police officers when a call comes over their radios: *Officer down, officer down.* I look at the two cops and say, "I don't know where that guy is, but you go bring him to me."

"I'm going, Mama," one of the cops says. "I'm going to bring him to you."

Two minutes later, three police squad cars pull up. I run outside, accompanied by two of my security officers. Hearing the eerie sound of all those sirens tells me that nothing good is going on. Seeing all those squad cars tells me that whatever happened is so bad, the police didn't have time to wait for an ambulance.

The wounded officer in the back of the squad car is Randy. He's been shot in the head. And he's unconscious.

"Randy, it's going to be okay. It's going to be okay."

But it isn't. Deep down, I know the outcome is going to be horrible. I can tell by the gunshot wound.

I take Randy into "recess"—our term for the code room where we bring very bad trauma victims so we can get things done quickly and determine whether the patient needs immediate surgery.

When an officer is hurt, a thousand cops cluster in the waiting rooms and outside the hospital. They don't listen to anybody; they do what they want to do. I stay there that night to make sure they remain outside the ER. I give them periodic updates.

Randy isn't going to make it. But we manage to keep him alive until his parents arrive so they can say goodbye.

Randy dies the next day.

I'm Irish Catholic—the fallen kind, mind you—and I believe that everything happens for a reason. I may not know that reason—may never know it—but there *is* a reason. Still, Randy's death shakes me. It's going to take me a long time to come to terms with it.

I get flowers delivered to me at the ER. I look at the card. *Thank you*, it says. *Detroit Police and State Police.*

There's something with cops. They know we're going to treat them well.

It's because we're a family. We all have our fights, and we don't agree on everything, but we all respect one another. They know our hospital is a safe haven, and that's the way I keep it.

JEAN ROGERS

Jean Rogers grew up outside of Philadelphia. She lives in Maryland and works as a pediatric nurse.

The psych patient pacing anxiously in front of the TV in the common room is thirteen years old and very, very big.

His name is Jason, and he's a new patient here at the private psychiatric hospital where I'm working part-time as a registered nurse. It's a Thursday night in 1998, and I'm twenty-five years old.

Here's what I know: Jason has been diagnosed with schizoaffective disorder (his symptoms include mania, hallucinations, and delusions) and another, more common disorder we see a lot here: oppositional defiant disorder, or ODD. This means Jason has, for more than six months, displayed extreme mood swings and angry, often violent outbursts that are generally directed at authority figures.

I've also observed three other qualities in Jason: he's quiet, calm, and creepy. But tonight, he seems very agitated.

I turn to another nurse and, my eyes on Jason, say, "What's going on?"

"It's Thursday night. 'Must See TV.'" The nurse catches my confused look and says, "*Friends* is about to come on."

(This was before Netflix and streaming, and *Friends* was at the height of its popularity. TV shows were broadcast at set times, so if you wanted to see your favorite show, you had to be sitting in front of your TV or you'd miss it.)

"And Jason," the nurse says, "is obsessed with Courteney Cox."

"How obsessed?"

"He believes Courteney Cox's character, Monica, is being persecuted by all the other characters on *Friends* and the actress really wants to kill her costars in real life but can't because she's a Hollywood star. He wants to kill them for her, especially Chandler. Jason really doesn't like Chandler."

I turn to Max, one of the techs, and say, "We should turn the TV off."

"Already way ahead of you."

Max leaves and shuts off the TV. Jason looks at Max the way he looks at me—at everyone. Not actually at you but *through* you. Jason is getting angry, and I'm thinking I'm going to have to call security, but Max manages to calm Jason down. He brings Jason back to his room.

Jason stays there and works on his journal. Doctors encourage patients to keep one, write down their thoughts and feelings. They even let Jason use a typewriter.

Two days later, Jason is sent to a state hospital. As we're cleaning his room, we find a composition notebook. It's his journal.

And it contains volumes of his thoughts on how he is going to kill all the characters on *Friends* in order to protect Courteney Cox. Jason goes into methodical and chilling detail about how he'll murder each one. What makes his journal even more disturbing is his method—Jason would begin writing by hand and then in midsentence start pasting in words and sentences he'd written on his typewriter. Then he would go back to writing by hand, this time lyrics from the Rolling Stones song "Time Is on My Side." Then more typing and more writing.

This kid is psychotic.

Seeing the murderous thoughts of someone so young is bone-chilling.

The journal ideas are very well thought out, and we wonder if Jason wanted us to find it. It's strange he would leave it behind.

If they ever let this kid out, I think, *I know one day I'll read about something awful he did.*

I'm working the three-to-eleven shift when one of our recently admitted patients, Kathy, this cute blond little eight-year-old who weighs probably forty pounds soaking wet, comes up to the nurse's desk. She can barely see over it.

"I want to play," she says to me.

"Sweetie, it's time to go to bed." We're very strict about bedtime because routine is important in order for children to get well.

Kathy pounds her fists on the desk. It's comical because she's so little. "I want to play," she says again.

"You have to go to bed."

This time she really pounds the desk. Her teeth are clenched and she's so angry, I'm waiting for flames to shoot out of her. *"I said I want to play."*

Her voice is like nothing I've ever heard in my entire life—guttural and demonic. It makes the hair on the back of my neck stand up.

I tell her no again but she won't go. Now I have to physically restrain her. I lock her in a bear hug, my legs around her legs. I'm holding her and she's fighting me with every fiber of her being.

The way she looks at me—the way she fights—I think she's possessed. No. I *know* she's possessed.

Kathy won't comply. We have to give her an injection. After we do, we put her in a padded room. The medicine kicks in, and, finally, she calms down and goes to sleep.

I'm a Christian, so I pray for her. *God, I don't know what this is. This is not my realm. This is You, God. You intervene.*

Years later, in private practice, I have an eight-year-old patient named Charlie. Samantha, a nurse with twenty-plus years of experience, goes into the examining room to get his vitals.

I'm speaking with the doctor in another room when Samantha screams for us.

The doctor and I go running in and stop short. We can't believe what we're seeing.

Charlie has the nurse in a choke hold.

We jump into the fray and separate them. The boy is abnormally strong, and he's seething at Samantha like a hellhound.

Samantha runs out of the room. I follow, leaving the doctor with the boy. I tell the boy's aunt and grandmother, who came here with him, what's happening, then send them back to the examining room.

Samantha is very, very frazzled when I find her.

"What happened?" I ask.

"I . . . I don't know, Jean. I was taking his blood pressure. He turned around, and then, when he saw this"—she points to the gold cross on her necklace—"he went straight for my throat. I couldn't fight him off. Jean, he was just so *strong*."

Unearthly screams fill the hall. I turn around and see the boy's aunt and grandmother. They have their arms looped around Charlie's arms. They're dragging him away, and the boy is fighting them with every bit of his strength. He's glaring at Samantha—at all of us—as he's walked out of the office.

Lord, I pray, thinking of my experience with Kathy, *this is not of this world. I know it's not.*

BOB HESSE

Bob Hesse taught combat medicine at West Point. He is the deputy chairman of the Curriculum and Examination Board for the United States Special Operations Command and the Special Forces medical adviser for the International Board of Specialty Certification.

At two in the morning, my fire pager goes off. I'm a full-time flight nurse and a part-time medical training officer with our small local fire department, and I often respond to medical emergency calls.

I'm told additional manpower is needed at a medical scene involving a sixteen-year-old girl giving birth at home. *Why isn't she at the hospital?* Then I'm told the address. It's out in the middle of nowhere, miles away from the nearest hospital.

I arrive, and I'm taken inside the house to a very small bedroom way in the back. The girl's mother is in there and is obviously distraught. Her daughter is lying on the floor between the bed and a wall. I can't see her—a medic is standing in front of me—but I can hear the girl sobbing.

The mother sees me and says, "I didn't know! I didn't know!"

"Oh my God," the medic says to me. "I'm so glad you're here."

"What's going on?"

The medic steps aside. The teenager is lying on her back with her legs spread open, and I can see the baby is breech. The baby's feet, instead of the head, came out first. The head is stuck in the birth canal.

A breech birth is an absolute emergency.

What's more, I see that the baby's chest, belly, and legs are blue and limp—and the baby appears to be very premature.

We need to get the girl someplace where we have room to work on her. I turn to the medic and say, "Get a cot in here, and let's move her to the ambulance."

As we bring the cot into the ambulance, I look at the young girl and say, "I need you to push."

"I didn't know I was pregnant."

"We'll talk about that later. Right now, I need you to push or your baby will die."

She does and, finally, gives birth to a twenty-four-week-gestation preemie boy, weighing mere ounces. The baby is limp, has no chest movement.

We begin ventilations and CPR immediately.

I have one of the medics start an IV on the mom, make sure she's okay, and as we connect a cardiac monitor to the baby, my thoughts turn to a six-month-old who came into the ER in cardiac arrest. In those situations, you have to have the mettle—and that's where I perform best, in completely chaotic environments. It's where I feel most at home.

I need to step into chaos again. I turn to a medic and say, "I'm going to see if I can tube this kid real quick, get him breathing. Give me a three-oh ET tube and a Mac one blade."

I'm able to intubate the preemie.

Through my skills and the grace of God, we manage to insert the tube. Still, I keep thinking, *I know this kid isn't going to survive. There's no way—*

"Oh my God," the medic says. "Look at the monitor."

We have a heartbeat. We run the preemie to the nearest hospital, which, fortunately, has a neonatal ICU.

The ride is a blur as we do multiple things to keep the preemie warm and alive.

The child makes it to the NICU.

A year and a half later, I run into the mother of the teenager who gave birth.

"You," she says, and she starts cussing me out. "Why didn't you let the baby die?"

"What are you talking about?"

"You were the one in the back of the ambulance who intubated my grandson."

"I still don't know what you're talking about."

"Yes, you do. You resuscitated my grandson, and you sentenced him to life on a breathing machine—and he wound up dying."

Then it hits me, what she's saying.

She's telling me I shouldn't have tried to save her grandson. That I should have just let him die.

I stare at her, absolutely and utterly astonished. I don't know what to say, but I'm thinking, *How can you say that?*

This isn't ancient Greece where they toss malformed kids off a cliff because they can't be Spartans. That's not how this goes.

She walks away.

It takes weeks for my anger to turn to empathy. I feel bad for the woman and her daughter, the loss the family went through when the child didn't survive.

I'm very self-critical. I review my performance minute by minute to see if there is anything I could have done differently.

Did I perform my best?

I did. There's no doubt in my mind.

I have no regrets about saving a life.

HONNA VANHOOZIER

Honna Vanhoozier grew up in Coppell, a suburb of Dallas, Texas. She studied nursing at Texas Tech and went to work in the ER right after graduation. Hana is currently an ER staff nurse at a level-one trauma facility in Dallas.

The ER nurse pushing a pregnant lady in a wheelchair says to me, "We're going to check her and make sure she's not crowning before we take her to L and D."

Not that long ago, we had a pregnant woman carried in on a stretcher. She was talking and then suddenly she stopped talking and coded. L and D got there, NICU got there, and we ended up doing an emergency C-section. I never saw one before, and there's a lot that goes on with it—lots of fluid and other stuff that is just gross. The entire time I was thinking, *I don't know how nurses work in labor and delivery. I am so glad I'm an ER nurse and don't have to see this every day.*

"Put her in the room right over there," I tell the nurse now.

I'm standing on the other side of the room starting to put on my gloves when the woman's baby comes out. It's literally falling out of her. The woman is sitting in the wheelchair and the baby is seconds away from hitting the floor.

I lunge across the room and, with bare hands, catch the baby.

The baby is a boy, and he's heavy, around ten or so pounds. I slowly get to my feet, careful not to slip on the wet floor, my hands and arms covered in all sorts of disgusting fluids. The wheelchair isn't close enough to the bed for me to place the baby there, especially because his umbilical cord is still attached to the placenta. The other nurse is staring at me.

"Wheelchair! Move the wheelchair!"

I find out this is the mom's ninth child, which explains why the baby just slipped right out of her. I'm cutting the cord and doing some other stuff when the ER doctor walks into the room.

"Um," he says, "who cut the cord?"

"I did," I reply.

"Oh. Okay. Do you guys need me in here?"

"No, I don't think so. I think we're good."

"Okay, bye."

I've seen a lot in the ER, but every once in a while, I'm hit with a surprise. One of the worst traumas I see involves a guy injured on a highway. He stepped out in front of a fast-moving semi. When he comes into the ER, he's mushy—every single bone completely broken. I can't understand how he's still alive.

In a case like this, when everything's broken, there's not much we can do for the patient. We start an IV and give him blood, but he ends up dying.

We have another patient, a male who was running from the police. He jumped a fence into someone's backyard and then figured that he'd rather go to the hospital than jail. His gaze landed on a lawn mower. He started it, flipped the mower on its side, and then, instead of shoving, say, his hand into the spinning blades, he decided to put in his head.

By the time he gets to us, it's clear that no amount of CPR will alter the outcome. This man is going to die. The doctor calls it, and the patient dies.

The top of the man's skull is flipped up, and his brain is completely exposed. It isn't bloody or anything. It's weird and yet absolutely beautiful.

But L and D is still gross. Just so gross.

I take care of a cop who's twenty-eight and newly married. He was in the boxing ring practicing for some kind of match between firefighters and police officers, got hit in the head, and collapsed.

He's covered in vomit when he arrives. We work hard on him. He has a bad head bleed, so we put him on a gurney and rush him straight to our neuro OR, which is a good distance from the ED, about ten minutes. Along the way, I keep thinking, *He's going to die. There's no way he's going to make it. This is awful.*

Two weeks later, he walks out of the hospital. Now he's back on the job. Every time we see each other, he gives me a big hug, and every time I think, *You were supposed to die. There's no way around it.*

We get another police officer in the ER. This man was riding a patrol bike and collapsed. We do CPR on him, get him back. He codes again. We do CPR on him again, bring him back, and again he codes.

This goes on for four hours.

He also should have died, but he didn't. Now he's back on the job and doing fine.

It's crazy how these things turn out sometimes.

Working in the ER has made me tougher. I see the world differently. When I board a plane or when I'm sitting in church, I look at people and wonder if one of them is about to code. Then I start to plan what I'll do: *Okay, that older woman sitting there in the middle of the church pew—if she codes, I'll have to get everyone out of the pew and pull them all off to the side, then I can bring the woman to that space right over there to the left of the altar and work on her. Yeah, that space is big enough. That'll do perfectly.*

This thinking isn't normal, but every good ER nurse I know does it.

I'm at a Halloween party at my apartment complex when a friend calls my cell. "I need you outside right now," she says, frantic. "I have a guy who's coding."

I'm dressed in a lion onesie and full lion makeup. She tells me where she is. I leave and run as fast I can through the parking garage, thinking, *Get there. You've got to get there.*

I bolt around a corner and find my friend doing CPR on a guy. I'm told someone called 911.

The man's neck, I notice, is quite floppy. I take over CPR, which is hard. It requires a lot of effort and you get tired very, very fast. You have to keep going, and when you do it right, sometimes you really do break ribs.

Paramedics take the man away. I find out later, while working at the hospital, that the man died. The night I found him, he had jumped off a balcony, which explains the floppy neck.

The great thing about nursing is that when your shift is over, you don't take home anything physical. I don't have reports or files or, like teachers, papers to grade. When I leave, I don't think or dwell on the things that happened that day. I go and work out and run errands.

If something really bad happens, I talk with my work friends, who are like counselors. I can bounce things off them because they understand, and then after a couple of days, I move on.

STEVEN COHEN

Steven Cohen grew up in Norwood, Massachusetts. He became a licensed practical nurse in 2008 and worked at a nursing home, a prison, and a state-run emergency/crisis services program. Steven joined the state's department of mental health as house manager of a group home for residents suffering from mental illness.

My nursing shift at the prison starts at three p.m. The first order of business is counting all the medications.

MCI-Norfolk, the largest prison in the Commonwealth of Massachusetts, has an all-male population of roughly fifteen hundred. In the prison pharmacy, we have over one hundred controlled substances, including narcotics, all under *very* strict count.

Not long ago, a nurse taped blister packs of Klonopin, Ativan, methadone, oxy, and Adderall to her waist and chest, underneath her shirt, just before the end of her shift. When she drove away from the prison, a few corrections officers tailed her. The nurse spotted them, abruptly stopped her car, got out, and started running. She reached a pond and ripped the tape off her body so she could dump the blister packs. That's where they tackled her.

It's crazy, what goes on inside this place. My shift is supposed to end at eleven, but most nights, work goes on until one in the morning.

After counting medications, I leave to administer the afternoon injections. One inmate, who was diagnosed with gender dysphoria, is a transgender woman on hormone therapy. She is in the process of suing the state to be transferred to MCI-Framingham, the state prison for women.

Today, she refuses her hormone injection. "Who cares?" she says. "The state pays for them anyway."

Each injection costs taxpayers three hundred and fifty dollars.

After a ten-minute break, I go to work the medication line, which can last anywhere from three to four hours. The prison is broken up into housing units. The inmates are herded, one unit at a time, to the nurses' station outside.

The nurses—I'm one of the few males—are separated from the inmates by a big bar. Corrections officers are with us, watching. Though the process is as regimented as a military operation, chaos always breaks through, especially on days like today when the weather is rainy and cold. No one is in a good mood.

And then it happens: I receive word that an inmate is coding—probably a heart attack or a stroke. With an inmate population this large, at least one person is going to code every day.

The line is shut down so that I can deal with the emergency, and when we pick back up, we're behind schedule. The nurse manager, though, wants everything done right, which is why I'm a bit obsessive-compulsive about making sure I give out the correct medications.

I'm not the quickest person to begin with, and with every minute standing outside in the freezing cold and rain, the inmates are getting more and more pissed off.

When I'm finished, Charlie, a corrections officer who's also a friend, says, "You do realize pretty much every inmate here wants to kill you."

It's a running joke between us. I play along. "And the corrections officers?"

"Yeah, they hate you too."

The prison's segregation unit houses ninety-eight maximum-security inmates. They're each in a small cell for twenty-three hours a day, and they get rec time for one hour. When I arrive with a female coworker to deliver their medications, they scream at us from their cells. Corrections officers accompany us wherever we go.

There's one inmate here, a guy named Jerry. He's serving forty years to life for driving the getaway car for someone who robbed and murdered a person. I think about Jerry a lot. He's a nice guy who I honestly believe is completely rehabilitated.

It does happen. Malcolm X was an inmate here back in the early 1950s. From a young age, he'd been involved in drug dealing, gambling, and prostitution rackets. He was arrested twice before coming to Boston, where he started burglarizing homes. He got caught and sentenced to eight to ten years. He paced around in his cell cursing God and the Bible so much that the other inmates called him "Satan."

Malcolm's life began to change when he went to the prison library. Equipped with only an eighth-grade education, he began studying the dictionary. Determined to educate himself, he took classes at the prison taught by instructors from Harvard, Emerson College, and Boston University. He even joined the prison's debate team and learned the art of crafting articulate arguments.

Jerry hadn't harmed anyone. He made one mistake, and now he'll be here for the rest of his life. It puts any difficulties in my own life in perspective.

My next patient is a well-known Mafia figure. The corrections officer opens the little metal door so I can hand him his meds.

"I want a Motrin," he says to me.

"You don't have an order for Motrin."

"Did your mother drop you on your head when you were a kid? Give me my Motrin or there'll be problems."

"Look, you don't have an order for it." If I give him one, I'll lose my job.

"Do you know who I am?"

As I turn to walk away, he screams, *"I'm in the Mafia. I know who you are and where you live, and I'm gonna get to you. I'll get to you. I'm going to kill you."*

I ignore him. I've had inmates yell at me before, although this is the first time I've been threatened.

I try hard not to take it personally. I try hard to put it into perspective by reminding myself that there are a *lot* of people who have it much worse than me, that I should feel blessed with what I have—and I have a lot. My faith in God helps.

*　　*　　*

Under no circumstances can someone who works in a prison form any sort of relationship with any of the inmates. They try to manipulate the shit out of the COs and the nurses, and they focus on female employees.

They say things like, "Can you do this thing for me? Just this one time, I promise." Do one thing for them—like give them a Motrin—and they'll ask for something else. If you say no to that, they'll say, "Well, you did that first thing for me, so I'll tell on you unless you do this other thing for me."

Sometimes the inmates' powers of persuasion get people into real trouble.

One day, a female coworker asks me, "How the hell could any female nurse get into a personal relationship with any of these guys?"

Two weeks later, she's caught sending love letters to an inmate.

KIMBERLY WAINWRIGHT-MORRISON

Kimberly Wainwright-Morrison grew up in Canadian, Texas, a little town northeast of Amarillo. She currently lives in Dallas and works as an ER nurse.

Luke is *really* gorgeous.

We've been dating for only a month. He's this goofy, good-looking bouncer, but he's not much of a conversationalist. I know he's not the guy for me.

Before we break up, Luke says something that changes the direction of my life—changes my entire being: "You know, you're pretty good at helping people. You should become a nurse."

I'm a college student at Texas Tech University. I came here to study journalism and then decided it wasn't for me. I've been thinking of changing my career path to teaching or writing, but Luke's words, for reasons I can't explain, make total sense to me.

I decide to go to a hospital-based nursing school in Lubbock. After I apply, I find a job at a beer store. The hours will work with my upcoming school schedule.

One day at work, before school has started, there's a car wreck right outside the store. I rush outside. A man and his son are badly hurt. I call 911. I watch the ambulances and EMTs and then the helicopter that arrives to transport the man and his son to the hospital, and I know, right in that moment, that my calling is to become an ER nurse.

The next day I call a trauma center and ask if I can get a job as an ER technician.

"I don't have any positions," the nurse manager tells me.

"I'll do anything. I'll change beds, clean, transport patients—*anything*. I really, really want to work there."

"I'm sorry, but I just don't have any positions right now."

I've always been a force-to-be-reckoned-with sort of person. I'm pretty insistent. We go back and forth, the woman and I, but she won't budge. "Look," I finally say. "I will lick the floor with my tongue if that's what you want me to do, but I need a job there."

There's a long pause.

Then the nurse manager clears her throat. "Can you start Monday?"

The ER is organized chaos.

It looks like a bunch of people running around, but when I watch closely, I start to recognize the moving parts that make the place function like a well-oiled machine. It's exhilarating, seeing these skilled professionals in action, seeing what they do.

I'm told that a guy in his mid-fifties is being rushed to the ER. He was driving a cement truck that hit a slick patch on the road and went over an overpass. The driver was crushed, but when the ambulance arrived, the EMTs found he still had a pulse. They bring him to us.

Watching the surgeons open the man's chest, seeing the nurses assisting with the surgical procedures—it's a lot to take in. And there's so much blood.

I find a wallet on the floor. I open it up. It belongs to the truck driver. It's filled with pictures of kids I'm assuming are his grandchildren.

This moment solidifies just how intense a career in the ER will be. Right then, I know my job will be more than just holding pressure on a wound to stop the bleeding. I'll be taking care of real lives—real people who have families who love them. Life, I realize, is very precious. It can be taken away at any moment.

KAREN MYNAR

Karen Mynar was born and raised in Canada. When she finished nursing school, she moved to Seattle and worked as an assistant director at a nursing home. She lives just outside of Dallas, Texas, and currently works at a level-one trauma center.

My patient knows he's going to die.

I'm pregnant with my youngest son and working the night shift on the stem-cell floor with oncology patients who are receiving experimental drugs.

Philip is twenty-one and has leukemia. Most of my patients, including Philip, are usually up all night, and I'm the only person they can talk to.

"I don't want to be by myself," Philip says now. "Would you come in and hang out with me?"

I'm doing paperwork for my patients' charts, and I can do that anywhere, so I bring the charts into his room, glad to keep him company. "What do you want to talk about?" I say. "Ask me any question. I'll tell you anything."

He asks me all sorts of questions: What does it feel like to be pregnant? What's it like when your children are born? What was it like when you got married?

There are so many things he wants to know.

I ask the sonogram tech to bring the ultrasound equipment to the room. She does a sono on my belly and shows Philip the images.

We talk about my pregnancy, about the fact that I'm having a boy, about hockey, about all kinds of stuff. It's a really profound moment for me because before this, he knew me only as the pregnant woman who worked the night shift and gave him his medicine.

He trusts me with some of his greatest fears and his disappointment that he's going to miss out on so much in life that he desperately wants to experience. As he talks, I keep thinking: *How in the world does this person trust me so much?*

Philip is slowly dying, and his family doesn't want to let him go. He's suffering and in so much pain that he's crying all the time. His family doesn't want us to stop giving him the experimental drugs because they know if we do, Philip will probably take his last breath and die.

The next week, Philip slips into a coma; shortly after that, he dies. I go home and cry and cry and cry. *I can't do this oncology thing anymore,* I tell myself, *because everybody dies.*

I move into critical care and emergency—and still see lots of people die.

My experience with Philip makes me realize that even though I connect with these patients only briefly, they are trusting me with their lives; they know that so much is in my hands. And I have to protect that. If they give me that look that says, *I trust you, I know you're going to do this for me,* it makes me go farther for them, go to the highest levels of exceeding their expectations just because I know that might be the only care they get.

A patient comes into the emergency department. He's been shot. It looks really bad. He's going to go to the OR, and there's a really good chance he isn't going to come out.

"Can I have a pen and a piece of paper?" he asks me. "If I don't make it out of surgery, I want to write a note to my wife."

I run and get the pen and paper. Because of his injuries, he can't write the letter himself, so he tells me what he wants to say, and I write it all down for him.

"Can you give that to my wife?" he asks.

I nod. "Give me her name and her number, all her information. I'll make sure she gets it."

He gives me her personal information and then he's rushed off to the OR. I go on with my shift.

I find out he makes it through surgery.

I visit him in his room two days later. His family is there. "Do you remember me?" I ask. "From the emergency department?"

He nods. "Yeah, I remember you."

"I have something that belongs to you."

He looks surprised when I pull out the note to his wife. "You still have that?" he says.

"Yeah."

He can't believe I've hung on to his note and actually tracked them down so I could make sure it got to his wife.

That stuff, he's probably thinking, only happens in movies.

"Would you like to give it to her?" I ask.

He nods. I hand him the note, and he gives it to her.

As I watch her read it and see the warm, tender expressions on their faces, my heart swells with pride and gratitude. Small, thrilling moments like this make every day of this tough job worth it.

KELLY SHOUSE

Kelly Shouse worked in environmental labs and taught seventh-grade science before entering nursing school with the goal of working in the ER. She now lives in Modesto, California.

As the daughter of a coroner, I grew up talking about dead people and nasty situations.

I still talk to my dad about the things I do and see in the ER—like today, when this little old nana comes in suffering from constipation. I perform what's called a digital disimpaction, meaning I stick my fingers up her rectum, and when I remove the hardened fecal stool, the woman goes, "Whoa, that feels great," and calls me her angel, which makes me laugh.

My mom doesn't like hearing gross stories. My girlfriend, who is a civilian, doesn't like me talking too much about my job either because she doesn't like how I laugh at things like this. "I'm sure that woman was in a lot of pain," she says to me. "You're not really empathetic."

I share these stories mostly with my dad and some close friends I work with because they get it. For people who work in the ER, humor is a key survival skill. It's not that I'm disrespecting a patient or disrespecting what I have to do or what the patient is going through; it's just that, as nurses, we have to find some humor in these situations or we'll all end up alcoholics or in the cuckoo house.

The coronavirus is really hitting Hispanic people hard, especially the ones who are overweight and diabetic. They're dying left and right. One heavyset Hispanic lady who comes into the ER starts bawling.

"You're putting your life at risk for us," she says. "You're saving our lives."

"This is what I do. This is my job."

"You saved my life. You're so special."

"I'm not special. I just know a little bit more about the human body than you do."

I have a patient who, for unknown reasons, can't breathe. We're going to intubate him.

He grabs my arm, looks me dead in the eye, and says, "I'm scared."

"I know. But we're going to take good care of you."

"No, I'm scared I'm gonna die."

"You're not going to die," I say. "You're going to be fine."

We put him under, and he dies.

The next morning, I'm eating my Cheerios and drinking a glass of red wine on the porch and just bawling and bawling when my mother calls.

"You need to talk to your father," she says, and she hands the phone to him.

I'm bawling so much I barely get through the story. He listens patiently.

"Kelly," he says gently after I'm finished. "This happens. It's okay."

My dad is more of a listener than a talker. He mostly just listens to me, which is all I need. But my experience with this patient is different. "I lied to him," I say. "I told him everything was going to be okay."

"You didn't lie to him. Everything *is* okay."

When my dad *does* talk, I listen. Still, I have a question to ask him. "What do you mean?"

"He went to the afterlife. I hear it's pretty awesome on that side."

I wipe my eyes.

"Kelly, you didn't lie to him. It's okay. He's in a better place."

When you're an ER nurse, you need a spiritual side. If you don't, the job will eat you alive.

LORI PALUMBO

Lori Palumbo grew up wanting to be Nurse Dixie McCall from the TV show Emergency! *and decided, in her thirties, to pursue a nursing degree. She lives and works in suburban Dallas–Fort Worth, Texas, and works as an ER nurse and a trauma resource nurse.*

I like to say a nurse is a jack-of-all-trades, master of none. Although trained nurses can quickly see what normal people can't, so that makes us masters of knowing when a situation is going to hit the fan.

People who come into the ER by ambulance go to what we call the "air traffic control desk," where we figure out where in the department to send them. I'm sitting near that desk when I see EMTs bring in a guy who is lying on the stretcher naked—which isn't strange; it happens all the time. He's facedown and making these really weird noises. We're told he collapsed after physical exertion and using drugs.

The naked guy's breathing is erratic. He's gone into what's

called agonal respirations, and at one point he doesn't take a breath for a good twenty seconds.

Yeah, I think, getting to my feet, *this isn't going to be good.*

The nurses who are getting ready to treat this guy are new. We call them "baby nurses" because they haven't racked up much time in the ER. It's not by any means a derogatory statement; they just don't have much experience.

"I'm going back with him," I say.

The older you get and the more experience you accumulate, the easier it becomes to know instantly in these types of situations what a patient's future holds. At fifty-two, I'm the oldest on the night shift. A lot of my coworkers are around thirty. I'm also older than at least two-thirds of the physicians. I'm old enough to have given birth to 98 percent of my coworkers. I'm at a different stage in my life. My kids are grown and getting married, about the age of these kids I work with who are also just starting their lives. I have a lot of life experience—and not just in nursing.

I start giving directions before we get the naked guy to the room. "Get me a crash cart. Notify the doctor we're coming, and get someone in the room from respiratory."

I'm taking the patient back when his heart stops.

We start compressions, get an IV in him, bag him to get oxygen in his lungs. Everybody starts coming in, and the doc is primarily concerned about intubation. I'm running the code with the drugs and doing chest compressions, the whole nine yards.

Compressions are taken over by another nurse. Drugs are handed to me, and the doctor intubates the patient. From the outside, it looks like chaos. It *is* chaos, but the organized kind, and I'm one of the ringmasters.

Despite our best efforts, the patient passes away. It turns out he was super-high on cocaine, which really didn't help.

We get a sixteen-year-old who coded out of the blue. He was playing volleyball with his family when he said he didn't feel good. Then he was on the ground and, essentially, dead.

Eventually, we're able to get him back. He's transferred to Children's Hospital.

This is going to be a horrible outcome, I tell myself. *This kid is going to be brain-dead.*

Through a team member who follows up on ER patients, I find out that the family is considering withdrawing care.

A few days later, I'm told the family has made the decision to let their son go.

Then, in what were to be the boy's final moments, something miraculous happens: he wakes up and starts pulling at his ET tube, trying to get it out of his throat.

I thought for sure he was dead. Now he's alive and on his way to a physical rehabilitation facility.

One of the things I've come to realize about myself is how well I can handle the chaos and the fast-moving pace of the ER and the death that comes with it — too often at the hands of other people. I've found a way to place each death in a box and put it up on a shelf. I take the boxes down every once in a while, unpack them, look at them, then put them back. I'm able to compartmentalize that stuff. I don't know if that makes me a twisted individual or just someone who's uniquely qualified to do this job.

But the main thing I've learned is that, as a nurse, you can do everything right, but in the end, God wins. If it's your time, then it's your time, no matter what we in the ER do.

MIKE HASTINGS

Mike Hastings manages the emergency department at Swedish Edmonds in Edmonds, Washington. He served as president of the International Emergency Nurses Association, an organization dedicated to providing tools, education, and resources to help medical professionals take care of people in their communities.

My boyhood dream in Independence, Missouri, is to get into law enforcement and become an FBI agent.

I'm sixteen and in the Boy Scouts when I meet a dad whose job sounds potentially even more exciting. He's a paramedic for the ambulance service in Kansas City. I ask if I can do a ride-along. I love the adrenaline rush of it so much that, when I'm eighteen, I get my EMT license.

Because of my age, insurance regulations prevent me from working for an ambulance service. I can, however, volunteer with the American Red Cross to do first aid at events. After getting my associate's degree, I transfer to a four-year institution to work on my bachelor's degree in criminal justice.

During that time, I'm on my own, a college kid living from paycheck to paycheck, working part-time jobs as a security officer for a shopping mall and at the communications center for our sheriff's department. We have some serious issues with the range of our radio system. If an officer makes a traffic stop in the southern part of the county and calls for help over the portable radio, there's a strong chance we won't receive the message. To fix that, we need to get the correct repeater system.

Some of the other communications officers and I decide to speak out about the need for an upgrade. I'm very vocal about it. I attend a county commissioner meeting to discuss the safety issue and how we can fix it. After the meeting is over, I'm fired from the sheriff's department.

I'm stunned. And crushed. My whole life has been about speaking up and helping people, and now I've been fired, not because of any wrongdoing on my part but because of politics—because a petty sheriff didn't like that I made him look bad.

I don't want any part of law enforcement.

I need to work, so I contact one of our county's rural EMS services and ask, "Do you by any chance have an immediate opening for an EMT?"

Thankfully, they do. Now I'm a city boy working in a rural environment, dealing with critical patients—like this man I've got inside the ambulance now. He was out alone and crashed his dirt bike. Somehow, he was able to crawl almost a mile back to his house, where he collapsed on his front doorstep.

He has cuts and abrasions from head to toe, and he's experiencing severe pain and some difficulty breathing, potentially related to the one or two ribs he seems to have broken. If he's bleeding internally—and there's a strong possibility that he is—he's going to need trauma care and, most likely, the expertise of a trauma surgeon.

The closest trauma hospital is forty-five minutes away. I'm worried; his prognosis is grim. I call for a helicopter, but there isn't a single one available. I call for a paramedic unit to come meet us en route to the hospital, but I'm told none will be able to get there fast enough.

Basically, we're on our own.

"I feel like I'm going to die," the man says to me in the back of the ambulance. "I can't breathe." The ambulance doesn't have advanced medical equipment, only basic first-aid tools and monitors. The guy driving is going as fast as he can.

"Don't let me die," he says.

I'm twenty-one years old and scared out of my mind.

"Please," he begs. "Please don't let me die."

This guy's life is in my hands, and there's almost nothing I can do for him. I feel totally and utterly helpless.

The best and only thing I can offer him is support. "You're not going to die," I tell him. "You're doing great, and we're doing everything we can. All you need to do is stay awake and breathe with me. That's it, stay with me and breathe. Just breathe."

When we reach the hospital, he's still awake and breathing.

We carry him inside on our backboard, and we accidentally leave it there. The ambulance can't do without this important piece of equipment. It turns out I have to be in the area the following day, so I volunteer to pick it up. I also want to ask about the man who got into the dirt-bike accident.

"He had some broken ribs, and he was also bleeding internally," I'm told. "We took him to the OR, stopped the bleeding. He's fine."

I'm glad—and relieved—by the positive outcome.

I work full-time for the ambulance service for several years. Then I decide I want something more—better pay and better hours, workplace conditions that don't involve spending hours outside in the rain and snow.

I decide to go to nursing school. When I graduate in 2004, I'm twenty-eight years old.

Nursing school doesn't teach you to be an ER nurse by any means. If you're lucky, you might get a couple of hours to shadow a nurse in the emergency department, but that's it.

In my senior year of nursing school, I'm fortunate to get a rotation at a level-one trauma center.

Nearly every day in the ER, I face life-and-death situations—and it's really difficult. The hardest part is adapting to the volume. Back when I was a paramedic, I treated one patient at a time. Now I'm learning to deal with multiple patients.

I discover quickly that I need to develop what I call a "bipolar approach" to nursing. I have to be able to witness the death of one patient and then instantly flip an internal switch and focus on the next patient's needs.

It's not easy.

There's no disputing that the emergency department is completely chaotic. But what the outside person would consider utter confusion is organized chaos to me. I thrive in this environment. I love constant action on multiple fronts, and I love dealing with the unknown.

One day, I'm told that two patients are being rushed to us, a mother and her eight-year-old daughter, both of whom were injured in an explosion at their residence. I don't know the details, don't need to—my focus is on the patients.

The mother comes in first. I'm assigned to her. I bring her into the trauma bay, and as I'm checking over her injuries, her daughter arrives. The girl is placed on the other side of the bay, and before they draw the curtain, I see that she is unconscious and badly burned.

The mom has burns too, but they're not as serious. She has superficial cuts to her extremities, and she's fully conscious. She knows her daughter is in here with her. She can't see her—the curtain is separating them—but she can hear the people working on her and she catches, as I do, words and snippets of conversation underneath all the noise:

Still unconscious.

Open her airway.

Intubate.

Her airway is severely burned.

The mom tries to get up. I gently place my hands on her shoulders, and as I help her back into a resting position, I say, "The team over there is doing the best they can. I promise you I'll bring you to your daughter soon, but you need to let me take care of you first."

She doesn't like it but she eventually agrees. As my team and I refocus on the mom, checking her for critical injuries, we hear a voice on the other side of the curtain say, "We've lost her pulse."

The mother tries to get up again. Again, I gently stop her.

"That's my daughter," she says.

"I know." I'm not a parent yet, but the emotional heart-ache she's facing really tears at me. "But you've been in a very serious accident. Stay here with me, okay? Squeeze my hand. That's it. Squeeze my hand, I'm right here with you."

Tears stand in her eyes. Her daughter is coding, and part of me so badly wants to pull back the curtain so she can see just how hard that team is working on saving her child. But I have no idea what's happening on the other side of the curtain, have no idea if they've opened her daughter's chest to reach her heart or performed some other medical procedure that will forever traumatize the mom if she sees it.

The daughter doesn't make it.

When we're sure the mother isn't critically injured, we wheel her stretcher over to her daughter's so she can hold her child's hand and say goodbye.

After we get patients stabilized, we send them off to the ICU or to a different hospital, so we often wonder what happened to this or that person.

But on those rare occasions when I get to know a patient's final outcome—those are the moments when it all comes full circle and leaves a lasting impact.

I'm working as the manager of a pediatric trauma center in Austin, Texas, when we're alerted to the case of a two-year-old who suffered an accidental gunshot wound to the chest. Unfortunately, by the time he reaches us, he has no pulse.

Two trauma surgeons and a cardiothoracic surgeon happen to be present. They have to open his chest, but they get the child's heart beating again. Three days later, the boy is running down the hospital hallway wearing a Superman cape.

Sometimes, the stars align.

CORINA STURGEON

Corina Sturgeon was born in El Paso, Texas. She worked for twelve years as a nurse in the emergency department and now works as a nurse practitioner.

The ER is where the shit happens.

When I was a burn tech at a Dallas hospital, it wasn't the wounds that got me; it was the abuse. In the span of nine months, I had one case where a two-year-old was placed in boiling water and another where a boy was lit on fire by the mother's boyfriend.

The one that hit me the hardest involved a four-year-old girl and her twenty-one-year-old mom, who was pregnant with her sixth child. For some reason, they were living in a hotel. The girl came in with burns all over her face, chest, and abdomen, supposedly from running into a space heater.

The story was fishy—the kid's hands weren't burned, and they should have been if the girl had, in fact, run into the space heater like the mom told the EMTs. The mother hadn't come into the ER with her daughter. She was nowhere to be found, and no one in the burn unit could get her on the phone.

The four-year-old ended up coding. Her heart stopped, and she was in multi-organ failure. We did CPR on her for two hours and finally got her back. The social worker on the burn unit kept trying to find the mother but didn't have any luck. The little girl coded again the next day and died.

Four days later, the mother finally got in touch with us. We explained what had happened to her daughter, and the mother asked to speak to the social worker. She wanted to see if the hospital would pay for the hotel where she was temporarily staying.

I went to my manager and said, "I can't do this."

"Have you ever thought about the emergency department?"

And now here I am, working in the ER at the same hospital where I was a burn-unit tech. It's my first day on the floor.

We're notified by BioTel, which is basically a command center for ambulances, that we're getting a trauma patient—a young woman who is nine months pregnant. She was on her way to the doctor's office when a drunk driver came across the median and hit her and her husband.

The ambulance brings the woman to us. We do everything we can to save her. We do an emergency C-section to save the baby.

They both die.

The husband comes in as we call the code on the mother and baby. The howling that comes out of him, watching him holding his baby and his wife—I know these sensory memories will never leave me.

* * *

Working in the ER is hard.

A homeless woman comes in covered in lice. The staff has to suit up. We take all of her belongings and triple-bag them. We coat her hair, her armpits, and her pubic area with RID. She's infested.

The EMTs are bringing us a nine-hundred-pound woman who had been lying on a mattress on the floor for such a long time that the mattress springs were embedded in her back. The paramedics, I'm told, had to cut off a portion of the mattress in order to get her out of her home and into the ambulance. She was lying on this mattress for so long that the skin on her back is stuck to the mattress material, and it will need to be surgically removed.

We see a lot of cases involving morbidly obese people, especially in the lower-income communities where families bring their relatives McDonald's and other fast food, then simply leave them lying on a mattress or couch. When a morbidly obese patient is too big to fit on an ambulance gurney, EMTs use tarps to bring him or her into the ER. We have to treat these patients on the floor.

This woman who's coming in, we're told, is covered in urine and feces. Room 17 in the ER is our decontamination room. It also has a door that's wide enough to accommodate her size. By the time the ambulance pulls up next to it, we're dressed in our hazmat gear.

As we do our best to clean her up, I find moldy food under her breast. She has roaches coming out from her body parts.

It's disgusting.

Then there's the issue of the embedded section of mattress

in her back. The springs are lodged in her skin, and because we don't have the necessary equipment to cut them, we call the fire department. They arrive with bolt cutters.

The woman is taken to surgery, where she's put under so doctors can remove the springs embedded in her back. She ends up dying.

A lot of teenagers, and even twelve-year-olds, are rushed into the ER because they overdosed on pills, often after attending "medicine cabinet" parties. Kids grab pills from parents' medicine cabinets, dump them into a bowl, then take a handful each. They don't know if they're taking heart medicine, pain meds, sedatives, or all of the above.

One girl—she was fourteen—came in unresponsive, not breathing. We coded her, got her back. But she was brain-dead. Her brain wasn't working and it will never work again, so now she's basically a vegetable.

She's brought into the ER every so often because she has a bad infection or a problem with her feeding tube.

Fourteen years old. She had her whole life ahead of her.

And then there are the psych patients. Some eat their shit and drink their pee. They smear shit all over themselves and all over the walls. One patient who's a regular in the ER has a colostomy bag. Out on the street, people pay him to have sex with his colostomy hole. He has drainage from STDs in his colostomy bag. When he gets pissed off at us, he slings his poop at the staff and police officers.

We have patients who punch us. We find guns on them, knives. We deal with prisoners. I deal with one who lunges at a cop, grabs his gun, and manages to get off a few shots before he's subdued. Luckily, no one is hurt.

I get another case, a nineteen-year-old who was remodeling a house with his twenty-one-year-old uncle. They were sanding hardwood floors, and the nineteen-year-old thought that instead of working in sections, it would be easier if he put the lacquer sealant over the entire floor and then buffed it.

Lacquer sealants exude extremely strong vapors and are highly flammable. One tiny spark was all it took for the nineteen-year-old and his uncle to be enveloped in a dangerous fire.

They arrive at the ER. The uncle's burns cover about 50 percent of his body. He's intubated and sedated so we can take him up to the burn ICU for wound debridement—the procedure for scraping off all the dead, burned skin.

The nineteen-year-old's burns cover 90 percent of his body—and he's still able to talk.

"I need to get hold of my mom," he says to me.

It's the end of my shift, but there's no way I'm leaving. I call his mom. After I explain who I am and why I'm calling, she tells me she's out of town and there's no way she or any of her son's family can get to the ER quickly.

I stand next to the nineteen-year-old and hold the phone for him while he tells his mother everything. He talks until he can't breathe anymore.

I stay with him until he dies.

I felt like I could serve the world as a nurse. But not in the ER. Not anymore. What I've seen, day in and day out, being called the B-word and the C-word, having shit thrown at me, people punching me and people bringing in guns—there's only so much trauma a person can see and take.

TOM O'HARA

Tom O'Hara grew up in Ticonderoga, New York. When he turned eighteen, he joined the navy and served all over the world, including in Afghanistan. Tom now works as an ER nurse at a level-one trauma center.

The hospital calls me at home. "If you can take a pay cut or if you want to go on a nice long vacation, let us know. Because the way things are going, we're getting to the point where we'll have to start furloughing people."

The reason is that COVID has led to widespread shutdowns, and hospitals are losing enormous sums of money. Surgeries—especially elective outpatient operations—are huge moneymakers for hospitals, but now everyone is staying at home and avoiding procedures they can put off until it's safe to go out again.

I feel sick to my stomach. I'm a relatively new nurse. I have only eight months of experience under my belt—and I have a mortgage and bills to pay. My wife and I just purchased a house we and our kids haven't even moved into yet. We're still living with my wife's parents.

For five months, I worked in the hospital's MICU, or medical intensive care unit. Now I'm working in med-surg (medical-surgical services), where I deal with a broad range of patients—those who are preparing for or recovering from surgery and those suffering from a wide assortment of medical issues. It's said that if you can make it in med-surg, you can make it anywhere in nursing.

"Do I have any options?" I ask the caller.

"Well, the company that owns our hospital owns others that are in COVID hot spots. They're swamped and really need extra hands. If you don't want to risk getting furloughed, you could volunteer to get redeployed. That's the best way to keep getting paid."

"I'll do it," I tell the guy. "I'll volunteer."

I'm sent to work in the ICU at a Chicago hospital.

My first day in the ICU in Chicago, two of the COVID patients code. Their hearts just stop.

Not a single one of the nurses looks concerned or surprised. They're not running around like this is an emergency. Their attitude is *Okay, we lost another one to COVID. What else is going on?*

It's like this COVID thing doesn't even faze them anymore.

As I start my shift, I sense that the odds of patients in the ICU surviving this disease are fifty-fifty.

One of my first patients is a young guy in his mid-thirties. He's walking and talking and wearing a nasal cannula, which is a tube that goes just below your nose and delivers supplemental oxygen.

He's still having trouble breathing, and the situation is deteriorating, so we swap the nasal cannula for a non-rebreather mask. The mask covers the patient's nose and mouth and is fitted with a reservoir bag that's filled with a high concentration of oxygen.

I crank up the flow. The patient seems to be doing okay.

Then he develops a new problem—he has to *actively* breathe, which means he has to work hard to take deep breaths, too hard to be able to sleep.

After two sleepless days and nights, he says, "I can't do it anymore. You need to put me on the machine."

We do.

He dies a day later.

It's confusing and frustrating how this virus affects everyone so differently.

And it wears on the people who are trying to treat it.

I went to nursing school with some of the nurses volunteering with me in Chicago. The camaraderie we have is unreal, the same as I experienced in the military—and these women are *tough*. They jump in to help with CPR or rolling a soiled, four-hundred-pound person.

Because I was in the service, I'm a bit more mentally prepared than most of the people working around me. When I went through combat training, we would have drills and then briefings where we were told what we would be up against. We were told some of us were going to die. I was young, eighteen. A hard charger full of piss and vinegar. I made peace with dying on the battlefield.

At the hospital, there aren't a bunch of salty combat vets preparing medical personnel for life in these virus hot spots.

I came back from Afghanistan with PTSD. I know the warning signs, and I can tell each one of these tough young women is lost in the fog of war. They're going up against an enemy no one fully understands—and they're losing. Seeing all of these deaths stack up day after day is making them question their abilities.

It's breaking them down.

I make sure to pull each nurse aside and ask how she's doing. Then I say, "Hey, when you get back home, promise me you'll talk to a counselor or another professional. If you don't, you're going to be a real hurting unit."

One night we get a transfer from another floor—a lady who had some recent surgeries, returned home, and caught COVID. When she came back to the hospital, her heart, I'm told, stopped several times. Because of COVID, she's also extremely septic—an advanced infection has taken over her body—and when she comes to the ICU, she's already intubated because she had stopped breathing on her own.

She's completely lifeless, but her heart is still beating.

The charge nurse comes to me and says, "Tom, I need your help with this."

A respiratory therapist is already inside the room, working the ventilator. When I look down at the patient, her eyes are rolled up into her head. She has incisions from a recent surgery running from her belly button to the middle of her chest. The incisions are surgically stapled, and they're bleeding and leaking yellow and green pus.

The woman is also a recent amputee; the lower portion

of both legs have been removed. Those incisions are also bleeding and leaking pus. Her bowels have let go, and she's completely covered in shit.

Her appearance shocks the hell out of me. And the charge nurse, this experienced woman who has been in the game for twenty-something years—she just loses it. I realize she called me in here for emotional support.

This patient is maybe a hundred twenty pounds. I work out—I can lift four hundred fifty pounds—but this lady is such deadweight that the three of us can barely move her into the ICU bed to get her cleaned up.

The whole process is nerve-racking.

By the end of my shift, this woman is somehow still alive.

But she's completely fucked up.

I've seen people with missing appendages before, and it's never bothered me. I saw a lot of things while fighting overseas. I mentally prepared myself for COVID before coming to Chicago, but for some reason, seeing what the virus did to this old lady, the state she was in—it just ends up breaking me.

I text my supervisor. The shit I saw tonight—I need the weekend off.

I completely get it, my supervisor replies.

That night, I drink Jameson straight out of the bottle. I'm not proud of that, but I'm in Chicago without my wife and kids, and I just feel so goddamn lonely.

I didn't have nightmares from my time in the service. Now I have nightmares every single night.

A month later, when I return home, I need to get tested before I can see my family. I call the employee health office at work and tell them where I've been, and they say I can't get tested because I don't have any symptoms.

"I haven't seen my family," I say. "I need to make sure I'm negative so I can see them."

"You don't have any symptoms, so we're not going to test you."

I try again, but it becomes clear that I'm on my own. It takes me a couple of days to find a place that will test me.

The COVID test comes back negative. I call my manager.

"When can you start?" she asks.

"What do you mean?"

"Working. When can you start working?"

"A month ago, you were asking people to take unpaid time off. You were going to furlough people."

"Things change."

I've been away from my family for a month straight. I worked nonstop, didn't have a support system of any kind, and saw people dying left and right. I'm wound up and on edge because I haven't had a moment to process everything that happened in Chicago.

I explain to her that when my tour in Afghanistan was over, the service sent us to Kuwait for five days to decompress, relax, and go through some mental-health workshops. When it comes to pain and suffering, people have different thresholds. Each person reacts differently to events, processes them differently. When I came back home to the States, the service gave us even more time to decompress because taking care of one's mental health and addressing any potential issues is critical.

"I hired you for forty hours a week," she says after I've finished.

"Chicago was like a war zone. I need—"

"Can you start tomorrow?"

At that moment I realize that my manager doesn't give two shits about me.

I go back to work the following day and start looking for another job. I'm okay mentally for a couple of weeks, and then I realize I'm suffering from PTSD—and for a reason I can't explain, it's far, far worse than what I experienced after I came back home from the war.

I'm in therapy now, and it's helping. I could easily go back to Afghanistan, but what I saw in Chicago...it still haunts me.

LOUISA PRATT

The daughter of a Marine, Louisa Pratt lived all over the United States as well as in Germany. Louisa now works as a staff nurse in a hospital emergency department.

Taking care of patients is not a Hollywood-glamorous career by any means. The day-to-day work is more gross than attractive. There wasn't a moment when I saw a nurse giving a patient a bed bath and thought, *This is the career I want.*

But I can see a value to meeting people at the most vulnerable periods in their lives. I see where nursing can take me, and where I want to go is either trauma or critical care.

As a postgraduate intern, I study and work twelve-hour shifts with another nurse. I'm working in a burn/trauma ICU that services a wide area, including Utah, Idaho, and parts of Montana and Nevada, when a patient in her early thirties is flown in from a hospital in Wyoming, intubated and heavily sedated.

The woman was caught in a field fire. Her salvage crops

caught fire, and the blaze escalated until she couldn't get out. Close to 90 percent of her body is burned.

Despite the extensive injuries, she's neurologically intact. Her family drives down, and we have a meeting where we discuss how ethical it would be to lighten her sedation in order to have a conversation with her.

The feeding tube we give her won't adhere to what's left of her skin, so we have to use surgical staples. I've never in my prior work at other ICUs encountered a burn so severe.

A recovery from such a traumatic burn, if it's even possible, involves years of multiple surgeries, physical therapy, and skin grafting. She'll be at high risk of infection, and she'll have to deal with unbelievable pain.

The parents tell us about their daughter, how earlier in her life she suffered from debilitating depression. I listen to them talk about all her struggles, and then the conversation turns to end-of-life care. I'm twenty-one, and this is the first time I've been involved in such a discussion.

The family decides to withdraw care. Now that I know about how this woman struggled, about all the things she went through, dying in a farm fire seems so unfair.

She ends up passing away.

The family wants to have a viewing at the chapel here in the hospital. The hospital approves it.

I will never forget wrapping up this now deceased person who was burned from head to toe. I will never forget any detail about the woman's physical body.

This whole concept of health-care workers as heroes—it doesn't fit with my experience. It's our job. It's what we signed up to do.

People in the military are heroes. I can't imagine running a code while being under fire or doing body recoveries in Haiti or in a massive catastrophe like 9/11. Those men and women are the heroes, the ones putting their lives on the line to save others. That's next-level bravery.

COURTNEY "C.J." ADAMS

Courtney "C.J." Adams is currently a nurse manager for medical-surgical ICU patients and progressive-care patients at a hospital in Ohio. She is also a captain and a flight nurse with the 167th Air Medical Evacuation Squadron.

ICU nursing is the epitome of the profession. The ICU treats the sickest of the sick, and traditionally, the nurses are the best of the best—they have to be in order to care for those patients.

Which makes me nervous, because although I have nursing experience, I don't yet have these critical-care skills.

My first hospital job as a nursing-school graduate was in neurology. That job gave me the opportunity to enhance my baseline skills and get comfortable being a nurse. I learned in depth about strokes and brain bleeds, but it was the dedication and support I gave to my patients that earned me a nomination for an Excellence in Patient Care award.

That job drove my interest in critical care. And now my new job in the ICU will help me reach my ultimate goal: becoming a flight nurse.

I had been working day shifts, but the hospital puts me on full-time at night. Night-shift nurses are a breed of their own. They sleep during the day, tend to hang out together, and share a strong morale. Every night-shift nurse knows what bars serve alcohol in the morning and which one is closest to the hospital. After rough nights, even our docs will go grab a drink with us.

We have a lot of rough nights.

Tonight, when I arrive for my shift, the charge nurse asks me to come into her office. She talks to me about a patient I dealt with yesterday—a Black woman who had a cardiac event that led to respiratory arrest. We put her on a ventilator, but we had a lot of trouble oxygenating her because her anatomy was atypical—she had a very small torso, so her lungs were compressed. We also ended up doing what's called targeted temperature management, where you cool a patient's body after a cardiac event to give the brain and body a chance to rest.

"We've rewarmed her and we're trying to minimize the damage, but it's not looking good," the charge nurse tells me. "Respiratory has been in there all day manually bagging her because we can't get the vent to cooperate. She's coded twice already. If she codes a third time, we think we're going to have to call it because there's just nothing else we can do."

All right, but why did you bring me into your office to tell me this? This is information I could easily have gotten from the day nurse's report.

"The problem," the charge nurse says, "is that the boyfriend is in there. He's causing a lot of drama, and we wanted to give you a heads-up."

Yesterday I talked to the woman's daughters but not the boyfriend. "Okay. Let me see what I can do."

I head to the nurses' station to speak to the day nurse and get the report on the patient. The station is directly across from this woman's room. The day nurse starts explaining about the ventilator's high-peak-pressure alarm. It keeps getting triggered because of the woman's respiratory problems, which is completely expected. The ventilator is on a default setting, and something as sensitive as a cough will make the alarm go off. Her readings, I can see on the monitor, are within appropriate limits.

Then, as if on cue, the ventilator alarm goes off. The boyfriend rushes out of the room and over to us.

The nurse I'm speaking to is white. I'm Black, like him, and his attention is fixed solely on me.

"She's dying," he says. "She's dying."

"Sir, it's okay," I say. "We know about the alarm—we expect it to go off."

"I'm telling you, she's *dying*."

"Sir, I had her last night, I'm very aware of her background. Anything that goes on in that room, I can see right here on the monitor. Let me finish getting the report and then I can give you a rundown of what's going on today."

"Okay." He's not happy about it, but he heads back into the room.

Thirty seconds later, as the nurse is giving me her report, the safety alarm goes off again. He comes back out and says she's dying again.

I cut the report short and take him back into the woman's room, hoping I can talk him off the ledge.

As I'm talking, I smell alcohol. *Is he drunk? And how did he get drunk?* From what I was told, he hadn't left the hospital all night.

Now I'm dealing with someone who is not only very anxious and agitated but also possibly hammered.

The alarm goes off again.

"See?" he says. "See, I *told* you."

"Sir, I need you to trust me. Like I said, the alarms are going to go off. We completely expect it, but I've got her. If anything changes, I will let you know. But right now, I need you to sit and be with her, hold her hand. Let me do my job so we can save her."

He slides his hand over my shoulder and draws me closer. He's five ten. I'm five one and tiny.

He looks down at me and says, "Can I stab you?"

I don't know what disturbs me more, the way he asked the weird yet frightening question so matter-of-factly or how he's now making slow stabbing motions against my chest.

He could kill me right now—and there's not a single thing I can do about it.

"Aww, I'm just kidding," he says. "Girl, you and me, we're going to be all right. I *know* you got this."

I'm frozen. I've been at work only ten minutes, and I can't believe this is actually happening.

I don't know what to say, but I have to say something to get out of here. "Okay. I got you. We're good. Let me finish getting the report, and we'll go from there."

I leave the room, and on my way back to the charge nurse's

office, I keep thinking, *What the hell just happened back there? Is he serious? What's going on?*

"Oh my God," the charge nurse says, horrified, after I tell her what went down.

"We need security, but don't have them barge into the room," I say.

"Why not?"

"Because all the security guards are middle-aged white men. This guy will lose his shit—and he's drunk. And if this woman dies while he's here, there's no telling what he'll do."

"We have to get him out of the hospital."

I realize that. "If I tell him that we've arranged a ride home and that security is going to escort him to that ride, that might work. Let's do this—you call security and have them on standby, and I'll go back and talk him down, get him to cooperate. Is that okay?"

She agrees. Reluctantly. My talking him down and getting him to leave the hospital without making a scene is the best outcome.

I go back to the room. The man is still there.

"Did you sleep here last night?" I ask.

"Yeah."

"I smell alcohol on your breath. Do you have any on you? Or were you guys up drinking and this is, you know, the aftermath?"

People come in drunk, especially in the ER, all the time. Having alcohol on the premises, however, is against hospital policy.

"We were drinking before," he says. "I don't have any alcohol on me." He buries his face in his hands. "This is my girl. If something happens to her, I don't know what I'll do."

If I don't handle this right, all of us are going to get screwed.

I sit down next to him. "I understand this is scary. I understand you have no idea what's going on. She's not out of the woods yet. I get it. If I were you, I'd be hammered-ass drunk too. But this is a hospital. Because you've got alcohol on your breath, and because of what's going on, we're going to get you a ride home."

He opens his mouth to speak. I stop him.

"I can't do my job if I'm also trying to manage you," I say in a gentle but firm tone. "I know it sucks, and I'm sorry, but if you want me to focus on taking good care of her and saving her life, then I can't be worrying about you."

"Oh, come on, man . . ."

"You want to do what's best for her, right?"

"I don't have a ride."

"Already taken care of. What's going to happen is that security is—"

"Don't you go bringing no police up here."

"This is security, not the police. They're aware of the situation, and they're going to make sure that you get your ride home and get some rest. Come on. I'll walk out with you."

He's still pissed, but he's okay with it. He doesn't resist.

After he's gone, we put the unit on lockdown and close the doors because we're pretty sure the patient is going to die, and I'm not sure how he's going to take it when he finds out.

As a nurse, I'm used to dealing with death. I'm blessed and grateful that my wife is also a nurse because she completely understands my job, and the support system we have, how we cope together, is amazing.

But this is the first time I'm afraid that my job could potentially get me killed.

The woman dies. The first few days, I'm worried her boyfriend is going to come back to the hospital. The ICU isn't locked down anymore. There's nothing stopping him from coming here.

Fortunately, he doesn't. We don't have any issues with him after that.

My next patient is a chronically sick eighty-something-year-old male who is suffering from a GI bleed. He's also on a ventilator.

Earlier in the day, he was put on an MTP, a massive transfusion protocol. By the time I arrive, the man has already been given multiple transfusions—packed red cells, cryoprecipitate, platelets, you name it—but the doctors can't stop the bleeding from his rectum.

"They took him to interventional radiology and scoped him to see where the bleeding was coming from," the nurse tells me as we're walking to his room. "They couldn't find an exact source, so they cauterized all of the arteries going to his rectum except one."

I know why. If they'd cauterized that last one, the patient would need a colostomy. "Did that do the trick?"

She shakes her head. "He's still bleeding."

"What about a CT scan?"

"It didn't find anything."

When I walk into the room, the man is lying on his back and getting another transfusion. The pad underneath him, though, is soaked with blood.

We have to see if the bleeding has stopped or if clotting has started. I help the nurse turn him onto his side.

In horror movies, when someone's limb is cut off, there's blood squirting everywhere—and that's what happens when we roll this man over. I have never seen so much fresh arterial blood spray out of someone before—especially from a rectum.

This man is going to bleed to death from his ass.

I call for one of the surgeons. Dr. Jones arrives and shoves his hand up the guy's butt.

"Okay," he says, "I think I found it."

He applies pressure. The bleeding slows down.

He removes his hand.

The bleeding starts again.

Again, he shoves his hand up there, and again he says, "All right, I think I found it." He applies pressure and slows the bleeding, but this time he doesn't remove his hand.

The patient, who has been given some light sedation because he's on a ventilator, drifts in and out of consciousness. He's becoming aware of what's happening.

I get on the phone and tell the on-call team that the patient needs to go back to the OR. Then I return to the room and start brainstorming about what we can place inside the man's rectum that will expand and hold pressure.

The patient is now well aware that he has a hand shoved up his ass and that he's bleeding. But because he's on a ventilator, he can't speak.

Everything we can think of inserting might cause more damage. The doctor can't remove his hand until the on-call surgical team is ready.

And he can't sit down. He has to stand at a certain angle in order to apply pressure.

"It is what it is," Dr. Jones says.

"Okay," I say. "I guess this is what we're doing tonight."

Dr. Jones stands there applying pressure for forty-five minutes. That's how long it takes to get the on-call team to the OR.

Dr. Jones's hand is cramped from all that time stuck inside the man's rectum. Someone else performs the surgery.

The source of the bleeding ends up being a hemorrhoid that somehow had arterial blood flow. The surgeon fixes the problem, and the patient stops bleeding.

For the next several years, every time I see Dr. Jones, I joke with him and say, "Hey, how's the hand?"

That night, I'm pretty sure, is the only time he ever saved someone's life by shoving his hand up the patient's ass and keeping it there for close to an hour.

The challenges I've faced on a regular basis as a critical-care nurse and now as a full-time nurse manager and a part-time flight nurse with the Air National Guard have definitely changed my outlook on life. I've learned that it's best to prepare for the worst. You have to be a little jaded to be a nurse. It's the way we save lives.

KARA BAUMAN

Kara Bauman grew up in Palm Springs, California. In high school, she worked as a candy striper in the pediatric unit. She went to the University of San Francisco on an ROTC scholarship and now works as a clinical educator at an emergency department.

My patient has a DNR, or "do not resuscitate," order. His wife is sitting at his bedside. He has multiple medical problems and he's unresponsive, and she's a mess, which is totally understandable given the circumstances.

"When he passes," the doctor tells me in the hall, "we're just going to let them have the time they need."

"Okay."

I don't want to leave this grieving woman alone. I go inside the room and stand next to her, watching the monitor.

A healthy heart keeps blood flowing through the body. Her husband has a dangerous irregular heartbeat, or arrhythmia, that affects the heart's ventricles. His heart goes into what's called ventricular fibrillation. In V-fib, the cardiac electrical system sends out the wrong signals, and the heart can't pump blood because the ventricles are quivering—or fibrillating. If it's not treated with medications, CPR, and electrical shock, V-fib usually leads to cardiac arrest and then death.

But he has a DNR because of all his other medical issues, so we can't intervene.

This is the end of the end.

I tense slightly. The woman senses it and says, "What's going on?"

"He's in his final moments. Please feel free to be with him."

She's crying, holding his hand. I place my hands on the woman's shoulders and just try to be her emotional support.

Her husband sneezes.

Oh my God. I watch what happens next on the monitor and then I rush to call the doctor.

"Our patient was in V-fib," I tell him. "He converted out of it by himself."

"What?"

"He sneezed and reset his heart."

"That . . . wait, that can't happen."

"Well, it did. He's starting to wake up."

The doctor comes to the room. He can't believe what he's seeing.

The wife is overjoyed. "It's a miracle! I knew it would happen if I prayed."

This man should not have lived. I have no medical explanation as to why he didn't die then, but I know I witnessed an amazing miracle. That's when I realized that it's God—not me—who decides who dies and who lives.

KAREN BENDER

Karen Bender grew up in Michigan's Metro Detroit area. She worked as a dental assistant for ten years and started pursuing a nursing career when her youngest child, Justine, was in kindergarten. Karen currently works as a registered nurse for Gift of Life, an organ-procurement organization for the state of Michigan.

The patient who's rushed into the trauma room is an older male with devastating injuries. He got behind the wheel of his vehicle drunk and caused a multi-car accident that killed two people.

In the trauma room, on the other side of the curtain, is a mother who just lost her child and her husband.

It's always difficult for me to find compassion and empathy for a drunk driver. What I feel mostly is anger. My job, though, is to treat patients. This drunk driver still needs medical care, and I have to provide it. I have to keep my emotions in check and put aside my judgment. I have to remain professional.

The police come into the trauma room. I know why they're here. Their suspect, the drunk driver, refused to blow in the Breathalyzer—which is his legal right.

"Is he under arrest?" I ask, referring to my patient.

They tell me he isn't.

"Then I need you to leave," I say. "We'll let you know when you can come back in."

The cops get angry. One says, "Are you protecting him? This guy who caused all this devastation?"

There are rules that need to be followed. If a suspect chooses not to blow in the Breathalyzer, the police need a warrant to get the suspect's blood drawn. They know the procedure.

They also know my job is to protect each patient. I need my patients to be honest with me. The police aren't held to any HIPAA laws, so if I ask a patient questions and the police are present, they can write down the whole conversation.

"Yes," I tell the cops, "I am protecting him because he has rights. That's my job. And if he's not under arrest, then you have no right to be in the trauma room."

"Oh, you like to protect drunk drivers, do you?"

Really? I want to say. *You know the rules.* And yet this cop is trying to bully me. He's questioning my integrity.

"I'm doing my job," I say. "I'll let you know when you can come in, but right now, you can't be here."

Soon after, the police bring me a warrant. Sometimes the warrant is illegible, and they get really mad when I tell them we need another copy faxed over.

Fortunately, this warrant is legible. Now I can legally draw the patient's blood to test for alcohol levels.

A cop brings me a blood-draw kit.

"This kit is open," I say.

"Well, yeah, I just opened it."

"But I didn't *see* you open it." The kit has to be sealed, and the cop has to break the seal in front of me. He *knows* this.

"That's the last one I have in my trunk," the cop says.

"Then you're going to have to find another one and open it in front of me."

"Oh, come on—"

"No," I say. "I have to follow the rules."

Nurses, cops, firefighters—we all go to the same bars and have after-shift cocktails; we all decompress and commiserate about the stuff we saw that day. We're here to help each other, but in the trauma room, you have to draw the line.

It's midnight when the hospital gets a radio call about a possible child-abuse case. The boy, who is two years old, has an altered level of consciousness, meaning he is in a coma-like state and won't wake up; the EMTs suspect the boy has suffered head trauma. They're bringing the child to us.

The call makes me think of my daughter. She's a new ER nurse, and she's pregnant with her first child. *When a child comes into the trauma room,* I've told her, *about ninety percent of the time it's because someone failed them. Always remember that. When you're at someone's house and they put a baby on the counter or they don't strap their kid in properly in a car seat or they don't make them wear a helmet when riding their bike—always be that person who speaks up.*

The two-year-old boy is a beautiful little towhead. But his body is limp. Floppy. He has what's called "raccooning"—bruising behind the ears and around the eyes. Raccooning occurs when a child is shaken or smacked on the back of the head really hard.

I feel sick.

We intubate the boy. We're all working diligently, calling pediatric intensive care and getting things done, when the police come into the trauma room.

"Is the mom under arrest?" I ask. We need to protect the child. We need to know who the child's support person is going to be.

"The mom is in custody," a cop says, "and we're trying to track down the father." The cop explains that the parents aren't together anymore.

Pediatric cases always hit me the hardest. The thought of an adult hitting a child is so upsetting—but I can't deal with that right now. I have to put my feelings away and focus on my job.

"The babysitter lives next door," the cop says. "She's the one who figured out something was wrong. She's here with her mom. Would it be possible for them to come in? They're extremely upset and want to see how he's doing."

The boy is stable, so I say, "Sure, okay."

The girl is fifteen and an emotional mess. She holds the little boy's hand and talks to him until he's whisked up to the ICU. It's obvious the girl cares deeply about him. I ask her what made her call 911.

"It just didn't feel right," she tells me.

"Could you please explain that?"

The girl tells me she got kind of a last-minute phone call from the boy's mother. *I just really need a break,* the mother told her. *He's already in bed—can you come over and babysit?*

It'll be an easy night for you. "I went over at ten at night," she tells me. "I made some popcorn and turned on the TV. Then I went upstairs to take a peek and that's when I got this feeling that something wasn't right."

She takes a deep breath to steady herself. "I turned on the hall light. I went in and saw he had this bruising on him, and he wasn't . . . his breathing wasn't right. I called my mom, and then she called 911."

If you hadn't done that, the boy would be dead.

I keep this thought to myself. I'm so awestruck by the conscientiousness of this fifteen-year-old. I don't think I would have been so aware at that age.

Kids falling off bikes or whatever, breaking their arms, getting stitches, bruises, and bumps—all that's part of a normal childhood. But children shouldn't get ejected from a car seat because somebody didn't buckle them in. They shouldn't be hit with such force that it alters their lives forever or, worse, kills them.

When you're a nurse, you're the family nurse, the neighborhood nurse—you're everyone's nurse, because nurses love taking care of people. We're the ones baking cookies for neighbors and checking on them. The couple who live next door to me are in their nineties and in phenomenal shape, but they still have health issues, and I know more about their medical conditions than their children do.

You get used to people always asking you medical questions. At a family gathering, my father starts asking me about erectile-dysfunction medications.

What? I want to say. *You're really asking me about this?*

ER nurses joke that we see more dicks than a prostitute does; the only difference is, we have better health insurance. I'm at a barbecue, and my brother's friend comes up to me, unzips his pants, and whips out his junk.

"Do you think this is an STD?" he asks.

"We're at a *barbecue*. Why are you showing me your dick?"

"Because I need to know if this is a rash or—"

"Maybe you should seek medical attention."

"I am. But I'd really appreciate it if you'd look and—"

"No," I say. "No, no, no. We're not doing this."

Nurses buy coffee for the policeman's wife who's been sitting by her husband's bedside. Because of budget cuts, there's no coffee in the break room, so we're the ones who go down to the cafeteria and buy coffee. Everything we do, inside and outside of the hospital, we do because we care—we just care.

JUSTINE KEEL

Justine Keel was five years old when her mother, Karen Bender, went to nursing school. Witnessing Karen's love of the job inspired Justine to follow her mother into a career as an ER nurse. She lives in the Metro Detroit area.

My mom is an ER nurse too. I call her from work and say, "I made a big mistake."

I always wanted to work in the emergency department. I wanted that level of craziness because . . . I don't know, something's broken in my head. But now that I'm in it, I realize I'm in way too deep.

"You've got to give yourself a year," she says.

A *year*? I've been an ER nurse for only a month, and I'm ready to quit.

"My first year," my mom says, "I came home and cried every day because I didn't know what I was doing and because I kept seeing so many bad things happen to people. Give yourself a year, and after that, you'll do it better."

I decide to stick it out. Months later, I'm working in triage when a couple in their late thirties come into the ER. They got into a fender bender yesterday and now the husband is having some chest pain, which isn't abnormal.

But I don't like the way this man looks. There's something more going on than his having been in a minor car accident. I decide to bring them back. We get him on the table for a CT scan.

The scan shows he has a balloon-shaped bulge in his aorta. It's an aortic aneurysm, and it's already ruptured. He's bleeding out and bleeding fast into his own body.

And there's nothing we can do to fix it. There's no way we can save him, although we'll try.

The woman stands alone, shell-shocked, watching everyone working around her husband. She's a wife and the mother of small children.

It triggers a memory—my mom calling home at the end of her shift and telling me I had to walk to school that day. When I asked why, she said, "I discharged a patient last night and I just found out she's been sitting in the waiting room for hours. She's ninety and has no one to pick her up, so I'm going to take her out to breakfast and then get her home."

There's nothing I can do for this woman's husband, but there are things I can do for her. I walk over and grab her hand.

The woman swallows. "He's not going to make it, is he?"

"No, he's not," I say gently. "But we have some time. Do you want your children here?"

"My mom has my kids."

"She can bring them in."

The woman thinks about it for a moment. "No," she says. "They're too little."

"Okay."

I speak to the doctors. "Can we make sure she has what she needs?"

They nod. We get the woman a chair so she can sit next to her husband's bed. She holds his hand. I do my best to comfort her. We all do.

If I can tell this wife that her husband is going to die—if I can help this poor woman who's watching her husband dying right now, knowing he isn't coming back home to her and their kids—if I can do this, then I can do anything.

At four a.m., a young woman in her twenties comes into the ER and starts pacing up and down the waiting room. I see her throw herself on the floor and start rolling around the way my toddler does.

What the heck is going on?

"Oh my God!" she screams. "I'm having a heart attack!"

Is this woman on drugs?

She gets up and somersaults across the waiting room.

Yeah, she's got to be on drugs. I get her vital signs. She's definitely not having a heart attack. "Did you take anything?" I ask her.

"No, I haven't taken anything."

I'm not buying it. "Okay," I say.

She starts rolling around and screaming again. I'm about to call security when she pops up and says, "That wasn't aspirin." Then she looks up at me. "The pill at the bottom of my purse. It wasn't an aspirin. I think it was ecstasy with some acid."

"What?"

She looks me dead in the eye. "You know, the pills you keep in the bottom of your bag for a good time?"

"I can't say I have acid or ecstasy in the bottom of my purse."

She's no longer listening to me. "I knew it," she says to herself. "I knew it." Then, to me: "Can I go home now?"

"Do you have a ride?"

"No."

"You just told me you took acid and ecstasy together, so unless you have someone who can give you a ride, I can't——"

"I'll call a cab."

She walks out. I stare after her, thinking, *What the hell just happened here?*

I take a break and check my phone. Daryl, one of my husband's buddies, has sent me a text: Is this herpes?

Below the text is a picture of his genitals.

This sort of thing has happened before. The last time was in my kitchen when one of my husband's friends exposed himself and asked for a diagnosis.

I text Daryl. Will you please warn me before you send a text like this?

Daryl texts back instantly. Your husband said you would look. Is this all right? Am I fine? Come on, Justine, tell me.

Parents come into the ER with a baby. I recognize them; they were here yesterday because their son, who is under a year old, had been suffering from vomiting and diarrhea from a normal GI bug.

The baby is floppy and unresponsive. We bring him back, get the doctor. We're trying to get an IV in the baby, but it's difficult, and he's going downhill fast.

"Why don't you have an IV in this kid yet?" the doctor barks even though the nurses are trying.

He starts yelling and keeps yelling to the point where the nurses are crying.

"You need to calm down," I tell the doctor. "We need to focus on this kid."

"What the fuck do you think I'm doing?"

"You're not doing this patient any good. You're scaring the nurses. You're making it so no one can do their job correctly. I'm not going to let you keep bullying people—"

"You're all ridiculous," he says to me and the room, "and you're going to let this kid die."

"You're done," I say, and leave.

I find a doctor I trust. "I know this is going to be a really uncomfortable situation," I say, "but the doc I have in the room is screaming at our nurses and making them so panicked that they can't do their job. I need you to come with me."

The doctor comes with me, and I bring him up to speed. We save the child.

My mom is my rock. I call her on my way home. It's six thirty in the morning, and when I hear her voice, I start sobbing. "Today sucked. Today really f-ing sucked. I hate the world, and I hate people."

"Okay. Tell me about it."

I run down my whole day. We talk, and after I'm finished, she says, "Would you like to go to breakfast? Do you want me to come and sit on the couch with you?"

"No, I feel better. I just needed to vent."

"Okay. Try and remember the good things you did today. Focus on the good."

She's right. And most days are not all bad. And every day there's something good I do for someone. That's what I hold on to—the good.

ALICE

Alice grew up in the South. She was twenty-eight when she decided to go to nursing school. She worked at a crisis center and at a treatment center and then as a traveling nurse. Alice now works in the ICU at a major hospital.

T he Natives," my dad says over the phone, "are alcoholics."
I'm about to report to my first nursing job. It's at a progressive care unit, or PCU, what we call an "ICU stepdown," meaning we treat people whose medical needs are more serious than what nurses handle on a regular hospital floor but not serious enough for the ICU. The PCU is in South Dakota, and our patients come from five Native American reservations.

"You'll see the Natives on the side of the road," my dad says. "These people have an intolerance to alcohol. They—"

"Dad, that's . . . so racist."

"I'm telling you the truth. Trying to prepare you. You've never been to a reservation. You'll see what I'm talking about when you get there."

I went to nursing school in South Dakota along with my friend Brad, who grew up on one of these reservations—the poorest one in the country, he tells me, and one of the poorest areas in the world. Brad gives me a tour.

I'm shocked at what I see.

The conditions are very third world. No electricity. Alley cats and stray dogs running everywhere, cars picked to pieces, mailboxes covered in bullet holes, and the homes, all of them, sprayed with graffiti, any valuable fixtures stripped and pawned. When Brad was growing up here, he tells me, his family had a lockbox for their mail so it wouldn't get stolen. This reservation also has one of the country's highest suicide rates.

These people have absolutely nothing.

I know what it's like to be judged. When I was a kid, I had a lot of orthopedic surgeries because of gymnastics injuries. I had no health insurance and my family couldn't afford to pay the huge hospital bills. I was treated like a piece of shit and I still remember the stigma of having bills that went into collections.

When I got so injured that I was forced to give up my dream of being a gymnast, I was lost. I became a hellion. My parents didn't know what to do with me. I didn't finish high school; I ended up getting my GED. I got a DWI at twenty-one and then, for the next ten years, I worked as a stripper at a gentleman's club in Miami, Florida. With my long blond hair and fake boobs, I look like a surgically enhanced Barbie doll.

And because of the way I look and my colorful past and the fact that I only have a GED, I'm constantly judged by people. A GED really isn't accepted as a high-school diploma, so I had to fight to get into nursing school in South Dakota. I told them I worked as a cocktail waitress at the gentleman's club, not as a stripper—and I got judged for that.

Which is why I made myself a promise long ago: I will never, under any circumstances, make someone feel like a piece of shit because they don't have health insurance or because they're homeless. I won't judge anyone based on what he or she does for work.

My job isn't to judge people. My job is to help them.

About 95 percent of the patients coming into the PCU are Native Americans living on the reservation. Alcoholism runs in their families, and a good majority have been drinking since they were young teenagers, so I see a lot of patients who are suffering from delirium tremens, or alcohol withdrawal. I have eighteen- and nineteen-year-olds suffering from end-stage liver disease.

There's a lot of physical and emotional abuse and an insane amount of sexual abuse and sex trafficking going on. Some of these people are simply doing the best they can, and some just don't know any better. It makes me realize how fortunate I am to have had such supportive parents.

I worked at a crisis center, so I have professional experience in mental health, alcoholism, and narcotic abuse. I also have personal experience in this area. When I was in nursing school, my bipolar brother tried to kill himself. Twice. Both times he was drinking a ton and overdosed by taking his entire ninety-day supply of clonazepam, a benzodiazepine that treats anxiety and panic disorder. Both times he almost died and both times he ended up in the ICU on a vent. He's lucky to be alive.

I sat with my brother for weeks and got to see everything that happens in an ICU. Watching the nurses, I decided that I wanted to work in an ICU someday.

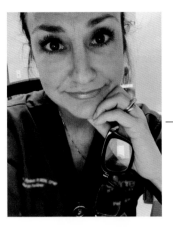 — Michelle Rylander

Jody A. Jamieson-Liana —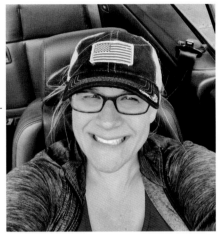

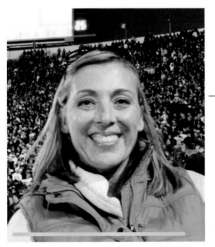 — Shannon Miller

Teneille Taylor —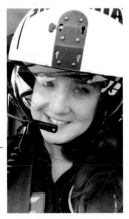

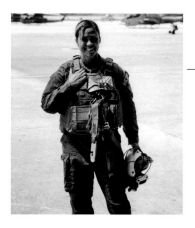
— Dominique Selby

Cyd Stephens —
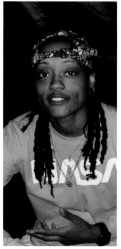

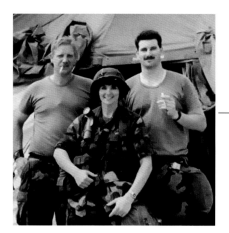
— Geraldine "Deenie" Laskey

Rosemary Baugh —
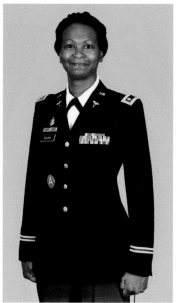

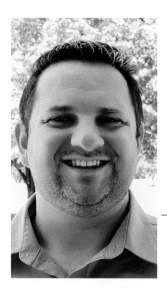
— Sebastian Berry

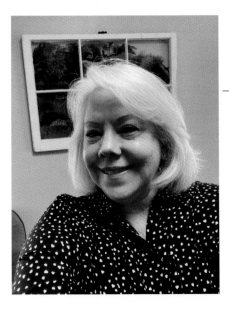

— Laura Van Syckle

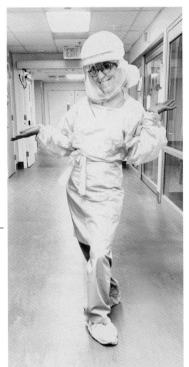

Tammi Bachecki —

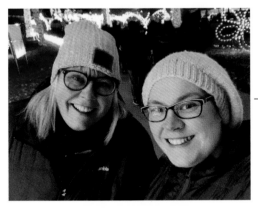

Karen Bender and
— Justine (Bender) Keel

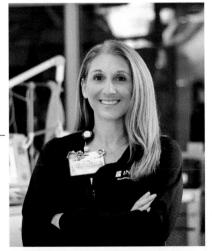

Kara Bauman —

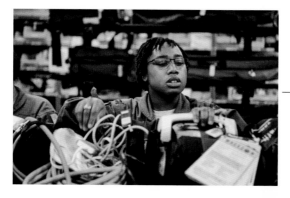

— Courtney "C.J." Adams

Louisa Pratt —

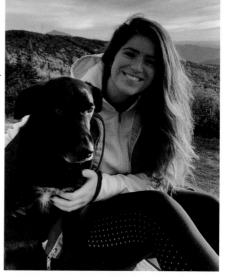

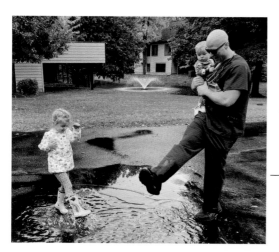

— Tom O'Hara

Corina Sturgeon —

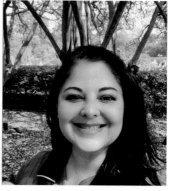

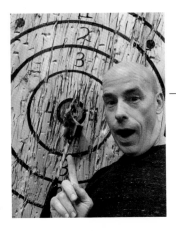 — Mike Hastings

Lori Palumbo —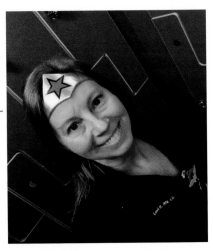

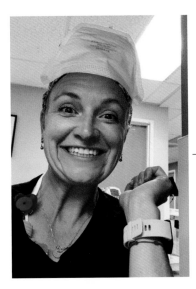 — Kelly Shouse

Karen Mynar —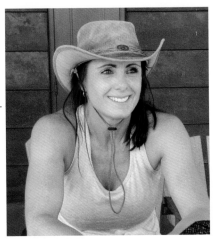

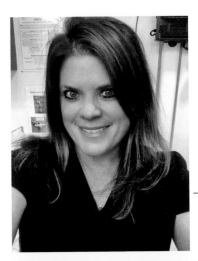 — Kimberly Wainwright-Morrison

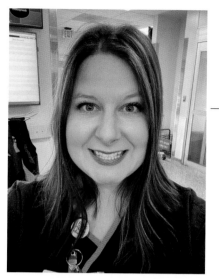

— Honna Vanhoozier

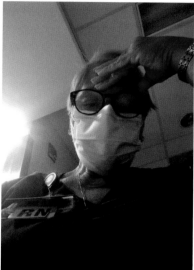

Colleen Champine —

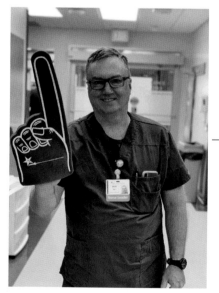

— Matt Bentley

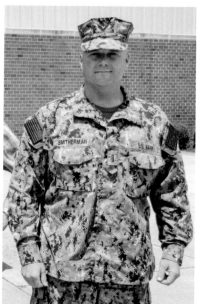

Jody Smitherman —

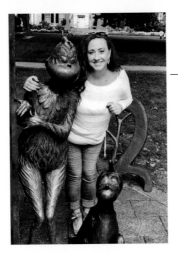 — Liz Martinez

John Antonelli —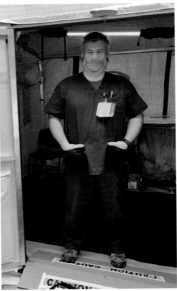

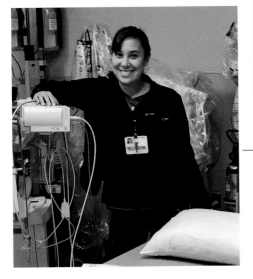 — Devyn Wells

Bethany Edmonson —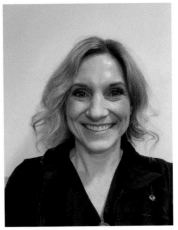

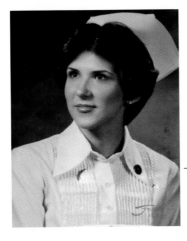 — Darlene Burke

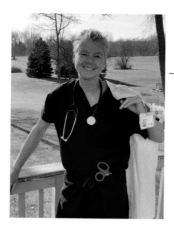 — Carol Rice

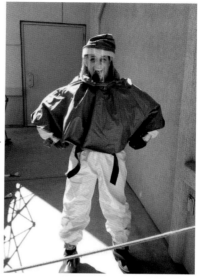

Andrea Perry —

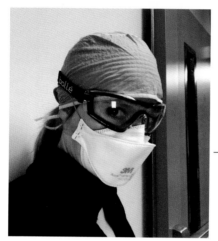 — Amber Richardson

Katie Quick —

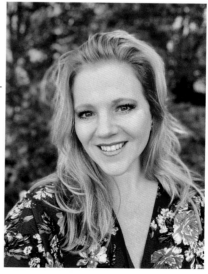

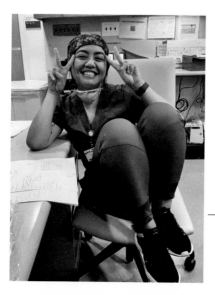 — Angela Parawan

My mental-health background helps me relate to these patients I'm treating in the PCU. Still, it's hard. Exhausting. And I'm not mentally prepared for some aspects of it.

Little old ladies in their nineties come in with UTIs so severe that they're delirious from infection. They punch me—it's amazing the strength some of them have—and a lot of them spit on me.

I get some patients who throw their own shit.

I'm so overwhelmed I can't stop crying.

The other nurses don't care. They're older. Burned out. They don't want to teach me anything. Instead of saying, *Hey, you're going to make mistakes. You need to pace yourself,* they say, "How can you be so stupid? Why can't you do anything right? Pick up the pace. You need to be faster." They don't know I was a stripper, but because of the way I look, they call me a stripper.

It's a very mean-girls, toxic work environment. No matter what I say or do, I can't do anything right in their eyes.

One thing is clear: I'm on my own.

One patient I get is a forty-year-old male with necrotizing pancreatitis, which means his pancreas is so infected it's dying. He's missing a good part of his leg from an above-the-knee amputation, the result of his uncontrolled diabetes. He's also had two transplants—a kidney and a pancreas—and he's on drugs that make him immunocompromised. He can't stop drinking, he's smoking three to four joints a day, and he's out of his mind because his body is polluted with toxins.

We have him in restraints—a vest that keeps his torso secured to the bed, wrist restraints that are secured to metal handles along the sides of the bed. His hands are covered with mitts to prevent him from tearing out the IV lines.

I'm trying to route a nasogastric, or NG, tube from his

nose to his stomach so I can give him his meds, but he keeps fighting me—violently twisting his head back and forth and kicking his legs because they aren't restrained. He's jacked on adrenaline, spitting at me and swearing, and his nose is bleeding from the fighting.

I need help. I leave and seek out a pair of big male nurses. I tell them what's going on and say, "I need your help. I need you to put the NG tube in him."

The two nurses follow me back into the room. We need to keep the patient as still as possible so the NG tube can be properly inserted.

One nurse gets behind the bed and presses down hard on the patient's shoulders. The other nurse stands on the patient's right side, holds the man's head still, and gets ready to insert the tube.

My job is to help keep the patient from flailing. His wrists are secured, but there's some looseness in the restraints.

I'm strong, I tell myself. *I work out. I've got this.*

I hold down his left wrist with one hand and then reach across the bed and grab his other wrist. I use the weight of my body to pin down his legs and keep him from thrashing.

The patient fights us with everything he's got.

His stump gets free, comes up, and hits me in the face. Cracks my chest and jaw; the sound is so loud that people down the hall hear it.

He hits me in the ribs—*crack*—and knocks the wind out of me.

I can barely breathe.

I'm going to be working here for eighteen months.

* * *

During that year and a half, I stop working out because I'm so exhausted. And depressed. On my days off, all I do is sleep, eat junk, and drink.

Finally, I decide I can't live this way anymore. I lean on friends and go to counseling. I start focusing on my health again. When I get overwhelmed, instead of drinking and eating junk food, I go to the gym or get on a bike, do something positive. I keep to this routine when I get jobs at other hospitals.

I work in several places, including the poorest sections of DC and Baltimore, but nothing can compare to the neglect and abuse I witnessed at the PCU in South Dakota.

My first ICU experience is during my orientation at a hospital in another state. The man who comes in is already intubated.

I read the doctor's notes. He is in his mid-fifties and retired. He and his wife were frequent travelers; they had just returned from a trip overseas and were preparing to head out to Vegas. They were at home having sex when he suffered a heart attack. The woman, a nurse, jumped into action and started doing chest compressions.

When the EMTs arrived, the woman was nude.

That's because she's a nurse. She knew it was more important to try to save her husband than to go and get dressed.

According to the notes, the patient had already had a bypass. When he had his heart attack at home, his body did not get an adequate supply of oxygen, resulting in hypoxia, which is a state of oxygen deprivation at the tissue level. Organs are affected within minutes. Based on what we're seeing, we're concerned that his brain was deprived of oxygen for so long that it's been severely damaged.

Once a day for two weeks, we give the man what's called a

"sedation holiday." We take him off sedation for a short period to see if he moves, if his eyes open or if his blood pressure increases. We're looking for signs of cognitive function coming back.

We don't find any encouraging signs.

After two weeks of hoping, the family decides to withdraw care. The man passes away. I stay with the man's wife that night, listening to her tell stories as she shares pictures of herself and her husband. Their kids.

In the days that follow, I can't stop thinking about the man and his wife and family. During those two weeks, his kids came in from all across the country and stayed at the ICU. Friends flew in from all over the world. The family basically lived at the hospital, and as I interacted with them, I was constantly amazed at the impact this man and his wife and kids had had on the world—how many people they'd touched and helped.

I want to have the same impact on the people I meet in my life.

I get a pediatric patient who's waiting for a lung transplant. Brenda has cystic fibrosis. Bad childhood—she was abused and put into the foster-care system—and she has no family. I work with her often and Brenda always asks for me. Consistent care helps patients, so the hospital grants her request.

While Brenda waits for her new lungs, she and I become close, and I help her through a few brushes with death. Transplants are expensive. She has a page on the website of the Children's Organ Transplant Association, which raises money for children and young adults who need lifesaving transplants.

I want to help raise money so Brenda can get her lung transplant. I get her written consent so I can share her information with my friends.

We raise a lot of money.

I'm not violating any HIPAA regulations, but I find out that I did violate hospital policy. The hospital, it seems, has strict social media rules. Still, I'm pissed. All I did was repost a page. Brenda's doctors did the exact same thing and didn't get any blowback.

I get suspended and put on administrative leave while the hospital decides what to do with me.

Hindsight is 20/20. I probably should have gone to HR to find out the proper protocol. I didn't stop to think about that. All I thought about was getting lungs for this girl who had lived her whole life with cystic fibrosis and was literally on the brink of death.

The hospital administrators realize it won't look good if word gets out that they fired a nurse who was helping a patient raise money for a medical procedure. I get to keep my job.

Brenda gets her lungs.

When Brenda leaves the hospital, she is going to need a lot of follow-up care and support. Families who have kids suffering from cystic fibrosis reach out to sponsor her. One family lives very close to the hospital.

Winter is coming, and I find out Brenda doesn't have any cold-weather clothes. I go through my closets, find everything that I don't need anymore. I deliver the items to Brenda to her hospital room, along with games and puzzles to keep her occupied.

The hospital doesn't like it when nurses get this close to their patients, but my human impulses won't rest until I help her, have a positive impact on her life.

I still keep in touch with Brenda on Instagram. I get to see her living her life, smiling, breathing air through her healthy lungs.

TAMMI BACHECKI

Tammi Bachecki grew up in the San Francisco Bay area. When she was a college senior, the care she saw nurses give her grandfather in his final illness inspired her to go into nursing. She lives in California and works in an intensive care unit.

A kid's been partying with his friends, drinking and snorting cocaine, and now he's come into the ER with a rapid heartbeat. He's seventeen.

We put him in the telemetry unit, where the vital signs of patients suffering from cardiac issues are constantly monitored.

I'm back at the nurses' station when I see, on the central monitor, that the teenager's heart rate is spiking. I run to his room.

His girlfriend is giving him a blow job.

Which explains why his heart rate surged.

This sort of thing has happened before. One of my

coworkers went to check on her patient and found him and his wife in bed having sex—which is just gross. Don't people realize that a hospital is a dirty place?

"For God's sake, really?" I say to the teenagers. "This is a hospital. What are you doing?"

They're kids. They aren't at all embarrassed—only annoyed at being interrupted. They get upset when I tell the girlfriend that she has to leave the hospital *now*.

Later, I tell a doctor what I saw.

He has an answer at the ready. "If he'd died, she would've been able to claim that she gives killer blow jobs."

I smile. "Well done."

JAMES THOMAS STENACK

James Thomas Stenack lives in West Virginia. For the past fifteen years, he's been an ER clinical insurance coordinator.

I'm seventeen years old and essentially living out of my car. I'm cold, tired, and hungry.

I grew up in the 1980s, and I was that kid no one paid attention to. My parents worked from sunup to sundown at their HVAC and electric business. My older sisters looked after me and my younger brother.

Now my parents are going through a divorce, and the family dynamics have just sort of disintegrated. I struggle to get through high school and graduate with a 2.0 GPA. I have no idea what I'm going to do with my life.

My girlfriend's dad is a full-bird colonel in the Air National Guard. She puts me in contact with him, and he puts me in contact with the recruiter.

I know absolutely nothing about the National Guard, but I take a standardized test called the Armed Services Vocational

Aptitude Battery, designed to show the positions in which you're most likely to succeed.

"You scored high enough on your ASVAB that you can go anywhere," the recruiter tells me. "What would you like to do?"

I have no idea, so he starts listing off possible careers. I stop him when he says "Air Evac," which is short for "aeromedical evacuation." Teams of specialists staff fixed-wing aircraft to transport seriously injured patients over long distances and at high altitudes.

"We have some openings there," the recruiter tells me.

It sounds interesting—and adaptable. I can take medical-related training and build on it, since the National Guard, at this time, offers 100 percent tuition reimbursement.

I jump on the opportunity. Three weeks later, I'm beginning basic training.

I apply for flight medic, but I'm placed in logistics. I'm not thrilled about it, but my thinking is that I can learn something and then transfer.

I look at firefighter and paramedic. I look into radiology. I start talking to flight nurses and flight medics.

They all ask me the same question: "If you're a paramedic or an EMT and you get hurt, what will you do then?"

What would I do? I don't have an answer. Those jobs, I know, require a lot of training—a significant investment in time.

"Nursing will offer you greater flexibility and more opportunities," one of them tells me. "Let's say you go the med-surg route and end up not liking it. You can go into the ICU. You can get into flight nursing. If you don't want to take care of patients, you can be a nurse paralegal. There are all kinds of different avenues."

It's the late 1990s, and there's a stigma associated with being a male nurse. If I go to nursing school, I'll have to fight that stigma from the very beginning of my career. That said, being a nurse will allow me to move laterally within the profession.

Nursing it is.

I start out as a cardiac-tech monitor, interpreting heart rhythms for twelve hours a day as I go through nursing school. Then I become a nursing secretary and enter orders and review patient charts.

The nurses are pretty loyal to one another—and they're great to me. I enjoy working with and for them. I spend so much time with them, they become like family.

A lieutenant colonel who is working as the ED director pulls me aside and says, "I know you're new to nursing, but you've got a year's experience. How about you come and work for me in the ER?"

In the ER, you have no idea what's going to come through the door—or when. Cardiac arrest, stroke, and trauma patients may all present within a few minutes.

I accept the job.

During my orientation period, we get a trauma patient, a fourteen-year-old boy. We work on him for quite some time, everyone trying really, really hard. Several hours later, we end up losing him.

I learn a lot watching the other nurses. But the biggest revelation to me is the boy's family.

Even though they've lost their loved one, they are so thankful to us for the care he received. We made such an impression that, years later, the boy's sister goes to nursing school and then comes to work for us. The boy's brother becomes an ED tech and works in our lab. All because of the care we gave their brother.

In that moment, I realize how fragile life is. And knowing that my actions can possibly help someone, maybe even save someone's life...I feel called to continue on a permanent basis.

As a new nurse, I often have to work the night shift. One night I come in at three a.m. and find all the nurses in the corner, giggling.

"What's so funny?"

"It's nothing," one of them says. "We need you to take care of the patient in room five."

"What's going on?"

"It's a long story. Just go in and see her."

Right then, I realize they're hazing me. I play along; I go into room 5 and pull back the curtain.

A young, thin woman wearing a G-string is lying on the bed. Three heavily made-up women in sky-high heels are with her. One of them says, "We work at the local strip club. Chardonnay"—she points to the woman lying down—"was dancing on the pole when she fell and hurt her neck."

Now I understand the nurses are definitely hazing me. I step away for a moment and collect myself because, even though this is serious, it's also funny. Then I do everything I can to help her.

Come to find out, she has a pretty serious injury—she fractured a vertebra in her neck. We have to send her out to another hospital.

Later, Chardonnay comes back to thank me. Every once in a while, she and her friends come by the hospital to bring us food and, sometimes, VIP passes to the strip club. It becomes a running joke in the ER. Anytime one of them comes in, the nurses will say to me, "Hey, your strippers are here to see you."

But there are serious moments too, like when a seventeen-year-old boy who's high on a synthetic stimulant known as bath salts charges at me. People on this drug are not only hallucinating, they're super-angry—and super-strong. He bites my neck and breaks a few ribs before his parents finally pull him off me.

We have shootings in the ER. Some stabbings.

Nursing school doesn't prepare you for that. It wasn't covered during orientation.

One night, a man gets jumped in the convenience store at a local gas station. His attackers hit him in the back of the head.

A head injury can cause patients to have angry, violent outbursts, and on top of that, he's already fired up about the whole situation. He's placed in room 27, which is directly across from the desk of the charge nurse.

Tonight, that's me. One floor nurse is busy dealing with a stroke patient, so I attend to the guy in room 27, help him get situated. He's wearing sweatpants, and every time I go check on him, every time I glance up at him from the charge nurse's desk, I see him reaching down his pants.

I don't pay any attention to it. That changes when one of my techs comes to me.

"This belongs to him," he says, and he hands me a concealed-carry permit.

All those times he's reaching down his pants, he could be trying to get his gun.

The tech and I go into the room. He doesn't have a gun in his hands, so we dive on him. He fights us as we wrestle him down, and the screaming and yelling attract the attention of the staff. They all come running to assist.

The gun, a nine-millimeter, is tucked in the waistband of his sweatpants, no holster. We manage to take it away. Fortunately, no one gets hurt.

That's not always the case. In one situation, a patient stabbed a correctional officer in the ER. We do everything we can to save him, but the officer dies.

I get another patient—a two-year-old girl who ends up passing away. We place her in a body bag, and because the ME can't come in and see her right away, I have to put her in the cooler.

I have daughters at home, one of them a two-year-old—a beautiful baby girl with blue eyes and long, curly hair. I'm a dad, and here I am being asked to put a child in the freezer.

Sometimes I come home upset, and my girls don't understand why. I try to put on a happy face for them, but usually I just want to be alone. Other times I want to be surrounded by a bunch of people. Sometimes I just want to talk to my wife, who can relate to my shifts in mood better than anyone because she is also a nurse.

Tonight, I just want to hug my girls a little bit tighter.

*　　*　　*

The patient who's rushed into the ER is a two-year-old boy who somehow got past the babysitter, left the house, and was viciously attacked by a pit bull. He's covered in blood. His face is mauled, and he's bleeding so much and so fast that he's a priority-one trauma. We assemble an entire team around him.

I work with others to clean up the blood so we can find out where he's bleeding from and try to stop it. As soon as we find one puncture wound and plug it, we find another puncture wound. We clean it and plug it up, then move on to the next one, and the next.

We have multiple IVs in him. We give him probably twice the amount of blood that a normal child has in his body to sustain him through transport to a children's hospital in DC.

But we have another problem—the weather is bad, and our helicopter doesn't have IFR capability.

As we work on the boy, we discuss taking him by ambulance. If we do that, because of all the heavy traffic, it's unlikely that he'll arrive in time for the docs there to save him. We decide it's best to keep him here with us.

As I'm suturing another wound on the boy, we get word that a flight crew has arrived. One of the paramedics, Brandon, is a good friend. He's also the brother of my former high-school girlfriend—the one whose father, the full-bird colonel, put me in touch with the National Guard recruiter.

"I've got room on this flight, and I'm going to need your help," Brandon says. "Do you want to go?"

I don't want to leave this kid. "Yeah, I'll go. I'll stay after we land so I can see him through."

We get word that we're clear to fly. We're on final approach, just two minutes out from the hospital, when the boy goes into full cardiac arrest.

Brandon and I work on the child the whole way down. When

we land, we get the boy into one of the trauma rooms. We're able to get him back. By the time I leave, they've given him more blood. He has a pulse, but he's intubated and in really bad shape.

Working in the ER, you don't normally hear what happens to your patients. You certainly don't hear what happens to patients who are transferred to other hospitals. But several weeks later, I hear that the boy has not only survived, he's made a good recovery.

He's alive because of the care and dedication of the ED staff and the supporting staff that came down from respiratory and trauma services. He's alive because of the passion of the helicopter crew working in coordination with West Virginia Medical Command. He's alive because of the quality care he received from experts at the children's hospital.

Nearly a hundred people came together just for this one child. It's a wonderful success story—maybe my biggest success story. I often reach for that bright memory, because most days are hard. The pressures day in and day out take a heavy toll.

There are different ways to decompress, and I like to mix them up. Maybe it's going for a run. Maybe it's going to the gym. Maybe it's taking a shower or sitting out in the hot tub and talking to my wife.

Or maybe it's saying, "Hey, kids, we're staying up late tonight. We're all going to sit together and watch a movie and eat some popcorn."

LAURA VAN SYCKLE

Laura Van Syckle was born in Binghamton, New York. She currently lives in Edgewater, Maryland, and works as an occupational-health nurse.

'm working at a California hospital when a young guy is brought into the ICU. His ID went missing at the site of his motorcycle accident, and all we know is his first name, Larry.

Larry, according to a CT scan, is brain-dead.

He lies in his bed, on a ventilator, alone, while the police try to locate his family.

Every twelve hours, a nurse goes into his room to do a neurological assessment. When I go in, I put my hand in his and say, "Larry, can you squeeze my hand?"

No response.

"Can you open your eyes?"

No response.

"Can you open your mouth?"

No response.

This goes on for ten days.

On the eleventh day, I go into Larry's room and ask him to squeeze my hand, then I run back to the nurses' station. "Larry squeezed my hand," I tell them.

"No. No way that happened."

I take the nurses to his room.

"Larry," I say, "can you squeeze my hand?"

He does.

One nurse runs to the other side of the bed. She places her hand in his and says, "Larry, squeeze this hand."

He does.

"Larry," I say, "can you open your eyes?"

He's not able to open his eyes, but he flashes his lashes.

We're jumping up and down, we're so excited. I start crying. Then we're all crying. We leave to call the neurologists.

Larry eventually wakes up and comes off the vent. He's twenty-nine years old. He's suffered some brain damage, but when he leaves us, he goes to a rehab center, where he learns to walk again.

Sometimes, miracles do happen.

PART THREE:

Flight Shift

ROBERT LASKEY

Robert Laskey was born in Michigan and raised in Ohio. As soon as he turned eighteen, he joined the army. He works as a flight nurse in multiple states.

I'm a flight nurse. I respond to accidents that happen all over Kentucky. My job is to make sure the patient doesn't die.

When a helicopter lands at a remote accident scene, there's no doctor or trauma team waiting; there's no lab or X-ray department. When the chopper lands, it's the flight nurse, a paramedic, and a bagful of medical equipment. We load the patient on board and fly to the big medical center in Lexington very, very quickly.

Only it doesn't always work out that well.

A guy in eastern Kentucky is driving his ATV when it breaks down, so he hooks it up to the trailer hitch of his buddy's beat-up pickup truck for a makeshift tow. This guy, who has had more than a little bit of alcohol, decides he's going to ride his ATV while it's being towed.

The vehicles are both traveling on the freeway at sixty-five miles per hour when the pickup truck makes a turn. The ATV does not.

I'm used to horrible car accidents where drivers and passengers have been absolutely mangled. I've seen a lot of farm accidents where people got caught in machinery and their limbs were ripped off. I've dealt with assaults and people with gunshot wounds. I've seen and dealt with pretty much everything.

When we land on the freeway, I see that the guy who was sitting on the ATV has left a very, very long skid mark of flesh, blood, and bone on the road. His body is barely intact. He's close to death.

I don't get emotional; I get to work. He's broken, and I'm going to fix his plumbing and keep him from dying, drop him off at the hospital, then go back to the base and make myself a chicken sandwich.

I get the patient on the aircraft. As we're giving him fluids and medications, he goes into cardiac arrest. I do chest compressions as we divert to the nearest hospital.

We can't revive him. He dies.

I see a lot of people in Kentucky who die from stupidity.

Some live through it. One guy had a broken gas gauge on his truck. It was dark out and he didn't have a flashlight, so after he took off the gas cap, he held a lighter up to the opening of the gas tank to see how much fuel he had. The gas fumes created a fireball, and he ended up with first- and second-degree burns to his chest, face, and hands. He lived, though he had some scarring. His lungs weren't damaged significantly because when he was hit by the fireball, he had the good fortune not to inhale. If he had, he probably would have died.

The stupid things people do are endless. A nineteen-year-old male who wants to be a YouTube star jumps off a roof, tries to grab a tree limb, misses, and breaks his back. A fifteen-year-old male makes a fire to burn Christmas wrapping paper and throws gas on it because the fire isn't big enough and winds up with second- and third-degree burns all over his body. He weighs four hundred pounds, and it takes the entire group of people on the ground—flight crew, firefighters, and cops—to pull this guy to the helicopter and load him onto the aircraft.

To this day, I'm amazed by adult stupidity that leads to hurting a child. We get a report about a four-year-old who's unconscious, and when we arrive the parents tell us they put their kid on an ATV without a helmet and let him ride it by himself. That kind of stupidity pisses me off—pisses off everyone on the team. It hurts us.

SEBASTIAN BERRY

Sebastian Berry grew up in Parkersburg, West Virginia, near the Ohio border. He currently lives in Utah, where he works as an ER nurse.

F ind a job that will never, ever go away," my father tells me. "A job that will always be needed."

I'm ten years old and my father is dying of lung cancer. He started smoking when he was fourteen.

My dad has lived a very hard life. He ran away from home when he was sixteen and bribed a judge with a five-dollar bill to write a letter saying that he was eighteen so he could enlist in the Marines. He's a World War II veteran.

I'm the man of the house. I take care of my father, doing his bed bath, changing his clothes and sheets. My mother gets up at two in the morning to start baking. She sells pastries and cold sandwiches out of the trunk of her car to businesses and private homes, and she works twelve-hour days.

We're very, very poor. Our house, which my father built with his own hands, has a dirt floor. To say I'm growing up in austere circumstances would be an understatement. The stereotypes you picture when you hear "West Virginia"—that's us.

"Those jobs," I ask my father, "what are they?"

"Anything to do with health care. People will always be sick." He pauses, thinking. "People will always be sick," he says again.

My father dies in 1985, when I'm twelve.

He's my first patient.

I'm a mediocre student in high school, and when I go to college, I'm more interested in the social scene than in attending class. I don't fail any classes, but I don't do as well as I should.

I enlist in the U.S. Army Reserve, in a military police company, because they need a medic. My training as an EMT will give me skills I can parlay into a job in civilian life.

In 2006, West Virginia Army National Guard troops are sent to the Radisson Hotel in El Paso, Texas, right near Fort Bliss. I'm part of a ragtag detachment made up of artillery men, cav scouts, MPs, and mechanics. We're going to run listening and observation posts so the U.S. Border Patrol agents can focus on actual fieldwork and apprehensions.

The people above me say, "Forget taking your aid bag. You won't be doing anything medical. You're doing eyes-and-ears missions." I take my aid bag with me anyway. If somebody gets hurt in the field, at the very least I've got Band-Aids and Tylenol.

We work with Border Patrol for months. The agents adopt us, and we become part of their family. We know one another's names and stories. We spend Thanksgiving and Christmas together.

In early May, Jim, an agent from the Border Patrol Search, Trauma, and Rescue Unit (BORSTAR), comes into my office and says, "Hey, do you have your aid bag?"

I nod. "I've always got it. I leave it here at the station. What's going on?"

"We're tracking a group of immigrants and we found one facedown in the sand. Can you help?"

I grab my aid bag. Outside the Border Patrol station, I bag ice and pack it into a cooler. We drive out to a place called Santa Teresa, New Mexico, about thirty minutes northwest of El Paso. Jim turns off the road and drives onto this large expanse of desert. In the distance, I see the lights of two, maybe three, Border Patrol trucks.

We approach a Hispanic woman lying on her back. She's barely breathing, unconscious, and nonresponsive. She's small, maybe all of five feet, and appears to be in her mid-forties. She is wearing multiple layers of clothes.

New Mexico gets pretty darn hot even in early summer. It's probably only 85 or 90 degrees but it feels like it's 110. I check the woman's radial pulse, on the inside of the wrist. Her pulse is what we call "thready"—really light, barely there.

I check her carotid pulse, in the neck, and it's equally thready.

The woman suddenly throws up her guts. I've never seen so much vomit come out of one person, and it's everywhere.

She's dying of heatstroke.

Jim, like me, is a field medic. I look at him and say, "We've got to get her cooled off."

"Agreed."

Border Patrol uses GMC Yukon Denalis, these big pickup trucks with covered utility beds. I grab three agents and say, "Move your trucks. Park them in L-shapes and give us some shade."

They move their trucks and tell us that the local EMS is on the way—fifteen, maybe twenty minutes out. Jim and I hustle the woman into the shade. While we've been at this for only a few minutes, I can feel time slowing down, like I'm moving through molasses.

"We've got to get her clothes off," Jim says.

We start peeling them off and quickly find she's wearing about four or five different layers of clothing. On top, she's got a long-sleeved sweatshirt, a long-sleeved T-shirt, a couple of short-sleeved shirts, and a bra. Same with the bottom—a couple of pairs of sweatpants, a pair of jeans, a pair of basketball shorts, and her underwear. She's wearing everything she owns so she can bring it with her to the States.

I look at Jim. "I've got some trauma scissors—do you have a pair?" He nods, and I say, "You get the top, I'll get the bottom."

She's wearing so many clothes, we have to make a couple of different passes to cut them all off. We have to get her "trauma naked" so we can do a full medical assessment, see if she has any injuries. We're assuming she has heatstroke, but we don't know for sure—maybe she was stabbed and is bleeding out into the sand, and we're just not seeing it.

We get her down to her bra and underwear. I don't see any injuries, so Jim and I take the heatstroke-treatment route.

"I've got the ice," I say. "Do you have anything in your bag?"

"I've got two liters of saline."

We pack her in ice, then I get a couple of IV lines going. I take her temperature underneath an armpit. It's 107. If I had done a rectal temperature, the reading would have been even higher.

There used to be these anti-drug TV commercials in the 1980s where a guy would hold up an egg and say, "This is your brain," then he'd crack open the egg and drop it into a hot frying pan and say, "This is your brain on drugs." That's what's happening to this woman right now—her brain is cooking.

We use ice and water to try and cool her down as quickly as possible. EMS shows up and takes her to the intensive care unit. I know she makes it there alive, but I don't know anything about her story until later, when Georgie Martinez, one of the supervisory agents in charge of the Santa Teresa station and a man I love dearly, fills me in.

"The woman didn't travel to the States alone," he tells me. "She was in a group of people." He knows this because of the amount of *foot sign*—their term for footprints in the sand—in the area. He tells me she was in a group of somewhere between ten and eighteen people.

I soon realize they left her in the desert to die because her "weakness" would compromise their ability to reach their destination quickly.

It breaks my heart. These people willfully abandoned a human being in the desert. What if she had kids? Maybe she sent her kids on with their dad or with what's called a coyote, a human smuggler.

It's my first experience with the evil people can do.

During my time in Texas, I've been applying to nursing schools. I get turned down at every one of them.

I decide to reapply to the nursing school at West Virginia

University, only this time when I write the essay about why I want to be a nurse, I include my laundry list of experiences and my time spent working at the border.

I know I'm not a very good student, I write. I know I have short-falls and shortcomings. What I do have is loads of experience. I'm currently the manager of our military clinic, and I've done things in my career that the brand-new students you're plucking right out of high school can only dream of trying. I have saved lives. I've held the hands of people as they died.

West Virginia rejects me.

I don't want to be in health care anymore.

In 2009, I get married, and my wife and I move to Utah. I start working for a health and fitness company headquartered in Logan. I start off at entry level and work my way up to middle management.

It's the deadest of dead-end jobs.

I'm still in the army reserve. One weekend while I'm driving to a drill at Camp Williams, just south of Salt Lake City, I see a highway billboard that says NO WAIT LIST. GET IN NOW. NIGHTINGALE COLLEGE SCHOOL OF NURSING. I later find out it's kind of a start-up nursing school, one of these for-profit colleges like ITT Tech and the University of Phoenix.

I apply and, living off student loans, eventually graduate. I'm a brand-new RN. I'm also flat broke, and my family is on welfare. My dream is to be an ER nurse, but my thinking is that I'll work anywhere. As long as I'm able to be a nurse, I don't care where I work.

In two and a half months, I put in something like 110 applications, from Logan all the way down to the South End of Salt Lake City. A community hospital calls me for an interview for a full-time position as an ER nurse.

The woman who interviews me gives me the job right on the spot.

The man comes to the registration window in the ER and says his belly hurts. That can mean anything from appendicitis to a bowel blockage to constipation. He's doubled over in pain.

I take him to a room and have him lie flat on the bed. As I press his stomach, checking for any obvious masses or tenderness, I start asking him questions: Did you eat something funny? Did you get hit in the stomach? When was the last time you went to the bathroom?

He seems to be answering truthfully, but I can tell something's off. I listen to his belly with a stethoscope and hear a rumble that's not a typical human bowel sound. I must not be using my professional "inside face" because he says, "Yeah, you heard that."

"I did. What's going on in there?"

"It's exactly what you think it is."

"Well, what do I think it is?"

Finally, he says it. Tells me he and his girlfriend were having a sexy time, got a little adventurous with the toys, and he ended up with a battery-powered vibrator stuck up his butt.

I press on his belly. I can feel the thing vibrating.

"Are you going to have to do surgery?" he asks.

"I'll have the ER physician come in and examine you. We're probably going to get an X-ray to find out just how far up this thing is, then the doctor can decide if he wants to try to fish it out of you here."

"That doesn't sound comfortable at all."

"You're already uncomfortable," I say. "How much more uncomfortable can it be to have someone put a hand in your butt to take something out of it?"

"Good point."

When I walk into the ER doctor's small office and tell him the story, I'm laughing so hard I'm crying. The doctor is thirty-six, around my age, and a jokester. We laugh a lot. In a deadpan, British-comedy way, he says, "Sebastian, this is really serious. You shouldn't be laughing."

Which only makes me laugh harder.

After I'm composed, we take the patient to X-ray, where we find out he's got a medium-large egg-shaped device stuck in his anus.

"I looked at your X-ray," the doctor tells him. "This . . . device hasn't traveled above your rectum. I think I can retrieve it. We'll use an anal dilator."

I come back with this hard plastic instrument that looks like a paper-towel roll; it has a flange on one end to keep the hole wide open. The dilator creates a big tunnel so we can see almost all the way into the patient's bowels. The guy's eyes get as big as dinner plates when he sees it.

We get the patient on his knees with his rear end high in the air. We lube up the dilator and insert it.

"This is not pleasant," the patient says.

"Yeah," the doctor replies. "I understand." He works for a bit and then turns to me and says, "I need the big forceps."

I come back with a pair of stainless-steel ring forceps that are roughly seven inches long.

"Oh yeah," the doctor says, "that'll do."

The doctor inserts the forceps into the anal dilator and grabs hold of this egg-shaped vibrator. When the doctor pulls it out, the amount of sound that comes out of this man's asshole is incredible—it's as if his butthole has been turned into a loudspeaker. It's so loud, the vibrating, clanging sound this toy makes while pinched between the forceps' metal rings.

"We're done here," the doctor tells the patient. Deadpan, he asks, "Do you want this back?"

"Yes," the man replies, and he takes his vibrator home with him.

My shift at the hospital is from six p.m. to six a.m. I got a lot of great orientation on the day shifts, and now, on my first night shift, I'm assigned as my preceptor, mentor, and role model an experienced nurse named Joe. He used to be a staff sergeant and a flight medic.

The nurses' station has a radio where we can hear all the pages for EMS. A page goes out for a car rollover with unrestrained passengers ejected from the vehicle, ages and number unknown.

EMS comes over the radio. "We're arrived on scene. We've got three passengers walking. One passenger awake, alert, but hurt."

But what kind of hurt? There's a big difference between "I've got some scratches and bumps and bruises" and "I can't feel my legs."

We're the closest hospital, so the patients will be coming to us. A couple of minutes later, we get an update from EMS over the radio. "This is going to be a trauma one. We need to call ahead."

A level-one trauma center provides the most comprehensive trauma care. Our hospital is small, with a six-bed emergency room. And we're a level-three center, so we don't have a trauma surgeon on-site, but our staff can stabilize patients before we transfer them to another hospital.

As an army flight medic, I've flown sick and hurt people. But this... this is all brand-new. I'm about to deal with a life-and-death situation here, on my first night. My butthole gets really tight, really fast. I look at Joe.

"You're going to be okay," he says, just as calm as can be. "You're going to be okay."

There is something about the competence of a calm leader, no matter the situation, that makes you feel like everything really is going to be okay. It's all going to be okay.

The ambulance arrives. A young girl between twelve and fourteen years old comes in with a neck collar and some bumps and bruises. For whatever reason, she wasn't wearing her seat belt. Car rolls over, ends up in a ditch, and she gets ejected.

She doesn't look terribly hurt, but she's writhing in pain.

This is my life now, I tell myself. *This is my life now.*

We take her to X-ray and find out she has a fractured skull and a closed femur fracture, which means the bone isn't poking through the skin. A broken femur can kill you. You can bleed to death. With a cracked skull, if the pressure inside your head increases too much, your brain herniates through the bottom of your skull, and then you're a vegetable. Either injury alone is dangerous enough, but when you combine them, the risk grows exponentially.

We end up sedating and intubating her to protect her

airway and her brain. Joe and another nurse do all the work while I act as a gopher, running for supplies.

I'm more than happy to do it.

In soldiering, when you get in intense situations, the fight-or-flight instinct kicks in. You have this huge adrenaline dump and you get either hyper-focused or hyper-scared. When the moment passes, you have to deal with a whole slew of emotions. We get the girl stabilized and loaded onto the helicopter, and once it flies away, all I can do is shake. I'm not scared or nervous; it's just the adrenaline wearing off.

I shake for nearly thirty minutes.

Joe, my preceptor, looks concerned. "Are you okay? Are you going to be all right?"

I recall the words of my dying father: *Find a job that will never, ever go away. A job that will always be needed.*

I've found a job that will always be needed.

And I feel needed.

"Yeah," I say, "I'm good."

And I am. This night cements it for me: Nursing is my calling. This is what I am meant to do. This is my home.

ROSEMARY BAUGH

Born and raised in Buffalo, New York, Lieutenant Colonel Rosemary Baugh was twenty-five years old, a firefighter and an EMT, when she enlisted in the military. After deploying to Bosnia, she went to nursing school and then focused on becoming an officer. She is stationed in Hawaii.

As an army nurse, you don't think about yourself. You have to put it away and do what you've got to do for the patient—and you always have to be strong because you're dealing with a life, and you have to take care of that life first.

You never know somebody's backstory. You're not dealing only with the present war. If you're a soldier, you might have things that are happening that you don't even realize.

Some medical people detach themselves from their patients. I can't do that. I have to be vulnerable and lay it all on the line. I am going to cry with patients, scream with them, get to know them. You have to be a little bit vulnerable to get through to your patients.

Still, when the military tells you what you're going to do, you do it. We have seven days to set up the first combat support hospital (CSH), which will consist of 296 beds, at a place called Camp Wolf, located in Kuwait.

The army drops us off in the middle of a desert. It's March of 2003. It's 130 degrees at midnight and there's nothing around us but brown sand.

I'm there with eighteen-, nineteen-, and twenty-year-old kids who just got out of nursing school, kids who now suddenly find themselves in another country, in the middle of a war zone, surrounded by, from what we've been told, weapons of mass destruction. Scud missiles shoot across the sky, and the U.S. military launches its own Patriot missiles to intercept them. We're constantly putting on our Mission-Oriented Protective Posture (MOPP) gear—gas mask, special gloves and boots, and clothing designed to be worn over our uniforms in the event of a chemical attack. We have to go into bunkers. I look at these kids and see panic and fear.

I'm much older than they are, and I have some maturity. I have a background in nursing; I'm a Christian and an officer. They look up to me and respect me. I try to bring some calmness to them in all this madness.

On day three, with the hospital nowhere near finished, we start receiving casualties.

When you're in a dire situation, there's no time for games. We're here to save the lives of our sons and daughters. Your background or what you've previously done doesn't matter.

When I'm told I'm going to work in the ICU even though I'm a cardiac nurse, I go, knowing it's literally going to be on-the-job training.

My first patient comes to me on the night of March 23, 2003, from Camp Pennsylvania. He's an army commander who has been shot several times in the back by, shockingly, one of his own soldiers, Sergeant Hasan Akbar. Akbar, a recent convert to Islam, believed that top commanders were conspiring against him because of his Muslim faith, so he switched off the generator at the camp, killing the power, and then, under cover of darkness, threw four hand grenades into the tents belonging to the 101st Airborne Division First Brigade Combat Team and his unit, the 326th Engineer Battalion. Both units were scheduled to invade Iraq the next day as part of Operation Iraqi Freedom. After the grenades exploded, he opened fire.

The commander doesn't make it. He's one of two people who die that night. Fourteen others, I come to find out, are wounded. In 2005, Akbar is sentenced to death by a military jury. He is still on death row at Fort Leavenworth, Kansas.

We also see and treat casualties from the local population. A car with a mother, father, and two children inside gets blown up. The father and the two children come to us, but for some reason, the mother is sent to a different hospital.

The little girl, who is three or four, loses an eye. The father has also suffered some injuries, but the two-year-old boy isn't hurt. They don't speak English. The boy is handicapped, and in that culture, the dads don't take care of children. That's the mother's role. We teach him how to change the son's diaper, turn him into a nurturer. The three of them stay with us, and we become like family. Eight months later, the mother is found, and the four of them are reunited.

A first sergeant who was a New York City policeman has a heart attack and has to go back to Germany. During 9/11, he got caught under something and now he suffers from PTSD, so we can't lie him down on a stretcher or strap him inside the plane. He's terrified of getting on the plane, so we have to sedate him.

I love taking care of people, which is why I got into the medical field. Because of the first sergeant's psychological issues, I fly with him to Germany.

When Fallujah falls, the statues are torn down. One lands on a tank and hits a soldier standing in the turret on the back of the head. He's paralyzed from the neck down. He's this really big Hispanic soldier, and he's crying.

"My wife is not going to want me anymore," he says, sobbing. "I'm useless."

In the Hispanic culture, the man is the head of the family. Hispanic men are really strong and proud. I tell someone to get his wife on the phone and bring the phone to me. I want him to talk to her *now*. I'm going to help this soldier get through this.

In 2006, I'm sent to a duty station in Landstuhl, Germany, where I take care of wounded soldiers in the trauma ICU. When they come off the bus, the first thing we do before we move them into the building is tell them, "You're here at a U.S. hospital. You're safe, you're in good hands, and we're going to take care of you."

Losing a soldier is the biggest fear for a nurse working a traumatic event. You're doing everything you can and thinking, *This is someone's son.* The survival rate of our patients is amazing. The ones we lose come to us either brain-dead or with so many catastrophic injuries that there's no way they're going to make it. For those patients, it's more about getting them to Landstuhl so we can fly in their families.

Nursing isn't just about passing out meds and fixing wounds; it's holistic. You have to deal with the mental and the spiritual—and the family. It's one package. Now you add to that devastating injuries that might end careers, even relationships.

Some of these soldiers are no longer in contact with a parent or parents or the ex-wife who remarried and is living a new life. Maybe they don't even see their kids.

One eighteen-year-old patient—I'll never forget his handsome face, his blue eyes and blond hair.

His name is Walt. He looks fine—no injury, no mangle or amputation—but he's brain-dead from a sniper shot to the head.

Walt's family is caught up in their own drama at home, and they opt not to come to Germany to visit their traumatically wounded son.

They decide to donate their son's organs. Since Walt's organs won't make it back to the States—we're just too far away—we partner with the German government to donate them locally.

That night, instead of going home, I go with Walt to the OR. I'm going to be with him when they harvest his organs, and I'm going to stay with him until he passes on.

I hold Walt's hand and sit close to his head in case he can hear me. I pray he can hear me.

"My name is Lieutenant Colonel Rosemary Baugh," I tell him as the surgeons prepare to remove his organs, which will go on to save lives. "You're not alone, Walt. Don't be afraid. I'll be with you the whole time. It's going to be okay."

GERALDINE "DEENIE" LASKEY

Geraldine "Deenie" Laskey grew up in a small town in Illinois. After going to nursing school, she joined the Wisconsin National Guard and was later deployed with the Thirteenth Evac to Desert Storm. Deenie retired after forty years of nursing, thirty of which were spent working in emergency settings. She lives in Wisconsin.

There are two rules of war," the psych nurse tells us as we mentally prepare for the ground war that is about to start.

She's a sweet lady with a calming presence. "The first rule is that people will die. The second rule is that you can't change rule number one."

I'm the captain, and I'm in charge of what's called a step-down unit—half ICU, half less acute patients. When you're a nurse in an ER in the States, you work your butt off and go home exhausted to your family, and then you can turn on a movie or order out and let somebody else cook for you. That's not possible when you're deployed, especially in the desert.

We're told to expect two thousand casualties immediately. I've got my ward set up; all the medical tools I could possibly need are stuck to the strips of tape hanging inside the tent.

My first patient is a soldier suffering an asthma attack from all the dust and sand kicked up by the forward movement of U.S. troops.

My ward ends up admitting prisoners of war because, for one thing, Saddam is putting schoolteachers and tradespeople on the front lines. They aren't really soldiers, but Saddam told them, "You're going to fight." They have no choice but to follow orders. When a young Iraqi kid protested, Saddam's men hung the kid's brother.

I end up taking care of the enemy instead of the coalition. Massive numbers of casualties flood the ER. I'm assigned to an Iraqi boy who can't be more than twenty, and he's screaming and screaming because he has a leg fracture and the bone is sticking out.

"This kid needs something for his pain," I say and ask for some morphine. I'm holding the syringe and bringing it to him when the kid goes ballistic on me. I give it to him in the thigh.

He ends up going to the OR. I visit him after surgery, taking a male translator with me. The kid is all smiles. I turn to the translator. "Ask him why he didn't want me to give him that shot."

The translator talks with the boy, then says to me, "He had been told by Saddam that if he was captured, we—the U.S.—were going to kill him. That's what he thought you were going to do with the syringe."

After more discussion between the two, the translator

tells me, "Saddam's people were ordered to kill anyone they captured."

A Humvee driver comes in from reconnaissance with some scrapes and minor injuries. He was wearing a helmet, which saved him from a sniper's bullet.

"Why don't we let you stay here for twenty-four hours," I tell him. "Don't go back out there. Take some time."

I tell all the soldiers this because they need time to decompress.

No one, soldier or medic, gets any relief.

It's day after day of twelve-hour shifts, getting calls in the middle of the night. At the ward, we're getting mortared almost every night, which means we've got to get out of bed, get to a bunker, go to the hospital for full accountability, and then, afterward, try to go back to bed.

The soldier shakes his head. "I got to get back out there. My soldiers need me."

It's what all the soldiers say.

Two weeks later, he's brought back to the ER. He's dead.

Another young soldier comes in with three of his limbs blown off by an IED. He's not going to live. Still, we try our best to save him. He dies.

My assistant, Matt, puts the soldier's body parts, which came in with him, in the body bag with him.

"How's his face?" I ask.

"It's not damaged at all."

I'm glad for that because I want his family to see him, not just his body parts.

Some of my medics are just babes in the woods. They don't have experience in trauma, have never seen these kinds of sights. I have to take them aside and say, "He would have died whether he was here or not, but having you here with him—that gave him hope."

Almost all of us are suffering from burnout. I was deployed to Kosovo, then went back for only a year and a half before I deployed to Iraq.

Being in life-and-death situations on a daily basis and then returning home to Wisconsin, where I've lived most of my life...I feel an internal shift that I find difficult to articulate, especially to my husband of thirty-six years. Over time, I come to realize that we want completely different things out of life—that we're on completely different paths.

I don't want to settle for mediocrity. I want something more because life is so incredibly short.

There's a personal cost to war. Each soldier pays a price—women especially. My price is my marriage. We decide to divorce.

It's incredibly painful, but it's the right thing for me.

And I'm hopeful.

Over the years, I keep asking myself: If I had to do it all over again, would I follow the same path? Would I still go into nursing?

The answer is always the same: I would do it all again. In a New York minute.

KAREN SPENCER

Karen Spencer was a senior in high school when 9/11 happened, and, unable to offer assistance at Ground Zero, she decided to study nursing. After graduating from college, she joined the army and deployed to Afghanistan in 2011. Karen lives in Oahu, Hawaii, where she works in a pediatric clinic at a military facility.

I t's the middle of the night when I land in Jalalabad. Everything's dark, but it's my first deployment and my senses are heightened. I've never heard a sound more vivid than the whirring of the Black Hawks.

That's when it hits me: This is real.

Up until this point, I've been working the flight line at Walter Reed Army Medical Center. Every Friday night, wounded warriors arrive needing treatment for amputations so fresh, they're guillotine-like.

Now I'm here in Afghanistan as part of a surgical forward team.

Two days later, a National Guard unit is hit. A first sergeant and two of his men were standing near a bomb. These are our first trauma cases, and when I hear they're coming, I'm thinking the worst, but they're not too bad. After we treat the first sergeant, he's allowed to return to duty.

I see him outside, smoking a cigarette. I join him, and we're joking around, blowing off some steam.

"Oh, man," he says, "they almost got me."

A week later, a soldier arrives covered in soot and blood. He's completely out of it. As we move him to a trauma bed, I hear what happened—this guy was standing very close to a suicide bomber who detonated his vest.

The soldier is in critical condition. We work to stabilize him.

The radiology tech shows an X-ray to the doctor. It's bad; the bones in the soldier's lower leg are shattered into hundreds of pieces. The soldier's radio also exploded and embedded a little coil and other parts in his soft tissue.

We don't have to intubate him, but we're going to have to evac him to Bagram. As I'm prepping him, I realize this soldier is the first sergeant I helped treat a week ago.

Later on, I'll find out that he lived. But in that moment, I'm experiencing my first gut check.

Four months later, in August, we're at the height of the anti-government uprisings known as the Arab Spring. It's fighting season, and it's intense. My medics and our soldiers are getting traumas nearly every day. We're also developing a good battle rhythm.

Our duties augmenting the forward surgical team's staff include dividing trauma teams for each bed, starting IVs, running labs, getting Foley catheters, all kinds of stuff. When we hear that an urgent 9 line—the army's version of a 911 call—is coming in, my medics take the field ambulance to pick up the wounded at the flight line.

The Black Hawk comes in fast and lands hard.

Oh, shit, this is going to be bad.

The field ambulance races back to the aid station. It busts a U-turn, and when the back doors fly open, I see the flight medic is performing chest compressions on a soldier on a litter. He's the one we have to get out first.

When I take over chest compressions, I realize I'm able to compress the soldier's chest to the extreme. *Oh my God, he has a flail chest.* This happens when three or more ribs are broken in two places, front and back, and become detached from the rest of the rib cage; part of the chest will move abnormally when the patient breathes. It's a common injury caused by severe blunt trauma.

It's also a catastrophic injury.

The soldier's blue eyes open and he tries to breathe. I help start an IV, take him to the OR, then go work on the Emergency Whole Blood Program—that's a tool we use to get fresh whole blood when we're running low on stored blood products. Prescreened people on the base who share the soldier's blood type are lining up to donate when I get the call that the soldier has died. When I walk back into the OR, it's eerily quiet, and there's blood everywhere. Nurses and techs are silently crying behind their face masks, the splash guards covering their eyes fogging up from their tears.

I knew his injuries were absolutely catastrophic. I knew that. Still, I don't understand why we weren't able to save him because up to this point, we've saved everyone. And now my patient is dead.

I don't cry. I need to be strong for my medics. There are really young kids here who haven't seen anything like this. I have to be strong for them. I have to comfort them.

I have a good amount of blood on me. I go back to my room, take a shower, then bury my face in my pillow and cry. When I return to work, the sorrow is still there, but now I draw on it like an inner reserve to make me try that much harder, work that much faster. We won't lose another soldier if I can help it.

MICHELLE

Michelle works as a flight nurse.

My patient's heart stops.

I'm brand-new to the ICU. It's my first job right out of nursing school, and every day is information overload. I go home in tears because every new case emphasizes how much I don't know, the gaps between a nursing-school education and treating patients in real time. And now my patient, who had open-heart surgery earlier in the day, is coding in the middle of the night.

I'm frightened and absolutely overwhelmed.

Oh my gosh, what have I gotten myself into?

I take a moment to remind myself that I had an amazing preceptor who trained me for this. I tell the team to get to work on the ABCs—airway, breathing, and circulation. It hasn't been all that long since I earned my Advanced Cardiovascular Life Support (ACLS) certification, and the details come back as I start doing chest compressions.

We finally get a pulse. Now that he's stabilized, I leave to use the phone.

I'm dreading the phone call I'm about to make.

When a patient has a cardiac event, you have to call the doctor or surgeon. In this case, I have to call the patient's surgeon—and surgeons, who are usually intimidating, do not like being woken up in the middle of the night. But my job is to advocate for the patient.

When the surgeon picks up the phone, I quickly find my voice. I explain that he needs to come in and assess his patient (who, it turns out, does have to go back to the OR).

When I hang up, I have this great big "aha" moment.

I can do this.

My next patient is a man with a colostomy bag who's suffering from gastrointestinal bleeding. He has diverticulitis and some other serious medical issues that have caused sections of his intestines to turn necrotic. He's had multiple surgeries in which these sections were removed and his intestines sewn back together. He keeps bleeding into his bag, and surgeons keep going in to "clip," or stem, the bleeding.

I'm with the surgeon when he has a care conference with the family. He explains why the patient can't endure another surgery. First, there's a strong chance he won't survive it. Second, the man has reached the limit for this type of intestinal surgery.

"Hopefully," the surgeon says, "we got it this time."

"And if you didn't?" a family member asks. "What then?"

"I'm afraid we've run out of options. If he starts bleeding again, there's nothing more we can do."

The family is beyond exhausted. We beg them to go home and get some rest. They reluctantly agree.

I have to go into the patient's room every fifteen to thirty minutes to check his colostomy bag for blood. Each time, I have to gown up and put on a mask and double-glove. In addition to his medical complications, he has an infection that can spread to other patients.

During one of my check-ins, I find bright red blood in his bag.

The bleeding has started again.

I have a bad feeling in the pit of my stomach. The patient sees the blood. I don't have to explain what this means. He knows.

I'm thinking of his family when he says, "How long do I have?"

"I don't know. Not long. You're bleeding pretty fast."

"I need you to help me write a letter."

I sit down next to his bed and start writing down his words—he's speaking as fast as he can, and he's crying. I'm crying too, and I'm trying to keep up with his words, trying to get them down perfectly. His family isn't here, and it gets me thinking about my parents.

I had just started nursing school when I got word that my parents had been in an accident. They were experienced motorcyclists, both riding their own bikes, when my dad suddenly hit a deer. My mom couldn't decelerate in time to avoid hitting my dad. She made the deliberate choice to "lay down the bike," meaning she purposely tipped the bike onto its side, which sent both her and the motorcycle into a high-speed skid across the road. An off-duty flight nurse who happened to be traveling in the opposite direction saw the accident and immediately called for a helicopter. He also called a nearby ambulance service.

My father lived, with minor injuries. My mother was flown to the nearest hospital, where it was found she had suffered a severe brain injury. She lasted about five months. During that time, I got to watch the amazing ER and ICU nurses care for my mom in inspiring, incredible ways. I made it my goal to work in every nursing area that had had some involvement in her care. I felt like I needed to give back—which is why, when I see how weak my patient is getting, I want to hold his hand. Without gloves.

I'm not supposed to take off any of my personal protective equipment. But gloves are impersonal—and this man is seconds away from passing. He needs human contact.

There are times when you've got to break the rules. I take off my mask, then my gloves. I get to hold his hand before he loses consciousness. He doesn't die with his family surrounding him, but he doesn't die alone.

I put my PPE in the proper containment receptacles and then wash my hands vigorously. After I'm fully sanitized, I type up the letter to give to his family.

I struggle with the guilt of encouraging them to go home and rest. Knowing that they missed that last moment with him is pretty tough, but I'm grateful that I was able to be with him. That moment, I know, will always be among the most memorable and rewarding of my nursing career.

Nursing, I realize, isn't just about medicine. It's also about making—and preserving—that human connection.

A farmer was on his tractor, running the attached harvester, when it malfunctioned. He got off the tractor, went to work fixing the equipment, and somehow got his hand caught in the machinery.

But there's more to the story. And it's chilling.

Farmers are paying exorbitant health-insurance premiums for limited coverage. On top of that, their crops are struggling, and farmers all over the state are barely making ends meet. This man is no exception. He's making financial sacrifices in order to keep up with his health-insurance payments. He doesn't have any savings.

He knows his insurance won't cover the staggering fees and hefty deductibles for an ambulance, hospital visit, and the other medical services he'll need for his hand injury. These fees, he's sure, will bankrupt him. If he calls his wife and explains what happened, she'll insist on calling for an ambulance.

He believes he has only one option—to amputate his hand himself. To do that, he'll have to use his pocketknife.

The pain is significant, but he coolly assesses the situation. His mangled fingers are caught, but his thumb has been spared, as has the lower part of his hand. All he has to do is saw away at the flesh just above his knuckles to free himself.

Still, the idea is horrifying. But there's no way he's going to call an ambulance. If he does that, he's convinced he'll lose the farm, everything he's worked and struggled for his entire life.

He takes a deep breath. *You can do this,* he tells himself.

He starts cutting. Keeps at it until he passes out.

When he regains consciousness, he goes back to work with the knife, then passes out again.

This goes on for hours.

When he finally manages to free himself, he wraps his mangled hand inside a towel and makes his way back home.

The wife sees what has happened and, despite all of his begging and pleading, calls an ambulance.

The farmer is nearly in shock when he arrives at the ER. He's also incredibly angry.

"I don't want to be here!" he keeps shouting. "I don't want any of this!"

EMTs, I'm told, have found the remnants of his hand and fingers. They've placed them in a cooler, and they're driving the cooler and his wife to the hospital.

"Just hurry up and cut off what's left of my hand. Amputate it, do whatever, but we're done here."

I try to calm him down. He keeps yelling that he doesn't want to be here, that his insurance won't cover this, that the fees and deductibles will destroy him financially. What I learn is that he basically wants us to let him die. That way, his wife will get the insurance money.

"If I live," he says, "the medical bills will crush us. We'll lose everything we have."

His wife arrives with the EMTs. Her husband is present when I explain to her that her husband should be flown to a surgical hospital, where surgeons will be able to reconnect his hand.

Her husband doesn't want to go there—he doesn't even want to be here. She goes to work trying to convince her husband to change his mind, to let us do everything possible not only to keep him alive but also to save his hand, and the entire time his anger is directed at me, as though I'm somehow coercing her to say this.

"I don't want any of this!" he screams at me. "Are you listening? *I don't want any of this.*"

The wife ends up convincing him to fly to the hospital for surgery.

I wait with the couple for the flight team to arrive. The farmer curses me out the entire time. "You've sunk us," he says to me as he's wheeled out. "Remember that. *You've sunk us.*"

He's right. Deep down, I know he's right. He isn't angry at me personally but at the medical system.

This event is a turning point. Even compassionate actions, I realize, have consequences. I urged the cardiac patient's family to get some rest, and they missed his last moments. The ICU nurses did the same with me when my mom was at the hospital. It was just a stroke of luck that I was able to say goodbye.

With the farmer, I urged him to undergo an expensive treatment on his hand. Fortunately, with my mother's situation, we had good health insurance. My family didn't go into debt. Some people, no matter how hard they work, can afford only a certain level of medical insurance. When catastrophe strikes, their insurance often fails them, and they're powerless as they try to navigate their way through our health-care system. Some can't afford insurance at all.

As I watch the helicopter fly away, I know there's a good chance that the farmer's accident might very well destroy him financially. It might very well cost him and his wife their farm.

CYD STEPHENS

For the past eleven years, Cyd Stephens has worked as an ER nurse and a flight nurse in California.

I work in a level-one trauma center, where I not only see the worst of the worst but have to deal with the world's worst thinkers.

Some of these people are addicts who also happen to be dumb. Others, for reasons I'll never understand, simply lack common sense.

Don't believe me?

A mom and dad come into the ER with their eleven-year-old daughter. The parents are high on meth. At home, the dad shoved something up his rectum, couldn't get it out, and ended up scooting his butt like a dog all around the house. Now he's here at the hospital, hollering in pain, and the mother is high and yelling at us. The daughter has the most unbothered look on her face, like she's been here at the

ER dealing with this exact same situation before. She opens a book and starts reading.

Two kids who live on a farm out in the country decide it would be funny to pee on an electric fence. They don't know that electricity transfers, so when the first kid takes a leak, the electric arc comes back, and his little genitals explode. He arrives at the ER absolutely burned, and we rush him into surgery to save what's left of his penis.

One lady, high on drugs, leaves her nine-month-old in a tub by himself. The kid drowns, and she tells the police, "I thought it could sit up."

A mother dumps boiling water on her three-year-old's lap because he was crying while she was making dinner.

Another mother, high on crack, decides to give her baby a bath. When her husband comes home and asks where the baby is, the mom says she doesn't know. Dad finds their child dead inside the washing machine.

These are the cases that take me by surprise and hit deep. After those nights, I get into the shower and cry. I log on to my social media accounts and message the people in my life, tell them, *I love y'all.*

In the beginning of my nursing career, I don't have an outlet other than my friends. There's a bar in Oklahoma that specifically caters to night-shifters. It opens early in the morning, and after a hard shift, we sometimes go there, hang out, and have a couple of drinks to decompress.

I don't think the average person can handle some of the things I've seen and heard. It takes a tender person to tell a mom that we did absolutely everything humanly and medically possible to save her baby and then leave to deal with a patient who is screaming at us to bring him his damn cup of water.

PTSD in health care is real and gets overlooked. It needs to be discussed, especially because a lot of us don't have families, friends, activities, hobbies, or outlets where we can find relief, and over time that causes a strain on our personal and professional relationships. I've been doing this for almost eleven years, and I need both hands to count the number of nurses, EMTs, paramedics, firefighters, and cops I know who have committed suicide.

I'm a licensed trauma flight nurse, and we get a lot of calls to deal with emergency situations in the rural parts of Oklahoma, where a lot of people live off the grid, without TV or running water. They often live together in these compound-type communities, the way cults do. The kids are homeschooled, everyone goes to church, and medical services are provided by someone in the compound. When there's a bad accident, however, we're called in.

Today, I'm responding to a call involving a fifteen-year-old girl who was riding her ATV, something she'd done a million times on her family's property. A couple of days ago, a storm came through. She's tearing down a path that's always clear, turns right, and suddenly smashes into a tree. She gets knocked out, and when she comes to, she's got a head injury and chest-wall contusions, possibly a collapsed lung.

I'm inside the helicopter, circling the property, which has Confederate flags and KKK symbols spray-painted in the yard and on the roof. There are swastikas spray-painted on cars, on top of the house (decorated in Christmas lights); someone even went to the trouble of cutting the grass in a certain way so there's a visible swastika pattern. It's so big I can see it up here in the air.

I'm a Black nurse. My pilot, Jackson, is Black, and Eddie, my paramedic, is white and gay and has earrings and pink hair.

Jackson looks at me and says, "Guys, we can decline."

He's concerned for our lives. This is how serious color is in this part of Oklahoma.

"I don't want to do it," Jackson goes on. "I will not land this helicopter unless you two tell me otherwise."

I've taken care of gunshot victims who have huge swastikas in the middle of their chests or on their foreheads. I've kept a lot of white supremacists alive on my watch, but it has always been in a hospital setting. This will be my first time treating someone behind enemy lines.

"I don't give a shit what color they are," I say. "I got called to do a job, and I'm going to do it. If things go awry once we're on the ground, then we can abort the mission. But I'm not going to refuse to help someone because of their biases."

I look to Eddie for his answer. He nods.

Jackson scopes out a landing spot in an open field. It's a good distance away from the compound. He radios the EMTs below where we're going to land and asks them to bring the ambulance to the main house.

The helicopter stays on the ground, its engine still running in case we need to leave quickly—and we might. As Eddie and I reach the compound, lugging our gear, I see a good dozen or more people are gathered outside on the porch and on the property. They're all wearing Confederate flag–emblazoned T-shirts and glaring at me because I'm Black.

I look right back at them and smile. *That's right. A Black woman is going to save your daughter's ass. You will forever be indebted to me. You're welcome.*

I'm hoping my presence will change their minds about Black people.

I doubt it.

As we walk to the ambulance, it's so quiet you can hear a pin drop. The people watching us don't say a word—there's no *Hey, how are you doing, thanks for coming, we really appreciate it.*

I open the back door of the ambulance and lock eyes with a big white guy with a thick, full beard sitting next to a teenage girl who's crying—the father and his daughter, I'm assuming. She's in pain and scared, and the fact that she's crying is a good sign. It means she's breathing okay. She seems both embarrassed by the situation and relieved that help is finally here.

The dad is heavily tattooed and wearing camo pants and a T-shirt with an American flag. He doesn't look relieved; he looks scared. I don't know if he's scared for his daughter or because he's face-to-face with a Black woman on his property. Maybe it's a little of both.

"You the dad?" I ask.

He doesn't answer. My gaze shifts to the EMT, a white guy dressed in jeans and cowboy boots. His name is Rick, and he's a volunteer firefighter. We've crossed paths before. He knows me and knows my heart.

He smirks because we both know that this situation is about to go one of two ways: either the father will let me treat his daughter or the father is going to get into it with me, and Rick will have to step in and defend me.

I take charge of the situation. "You can put your heart at ease," I tell the dad. "Between me and this guy standing next to me, you've got probably the best nurse and flight medic flying the skies of Oklahoma right now." I smile and put my hand on his shoulder. "Your daughter is going to be just fine. You'll be able to come and see her first thing tomorrow."

I look to the girl. "Have you been on a helicopter before?"

"No."

"Let's go for a ride."

This is it, the moment of truth. The father can refuse medical care. He can refuse to let his daughter go with a Black nurse and a gay paramedic, or he can let us do our job. He has to make that decision right now.

The dad's hard gaze lingers on me for a moment. Then he turns his head slowly to his daughter, and I tense, expecting the worst.

He nods his consent.

I put out my hand.

The father shakes it but doesn't say a word.

The next morning, a white supremacist gets released from jail in rural Oklahoma and decides to go explore someone's property.

The homeowner is there. He sees a man looking around his property, and he gets his gun. When the guy decides to let himself into the homeowner's truck—maybe to steal it, maybe to get warm because it's cold out—the homeowner confronts him. Some sort of altercation ensues, and the former inmate is shot.

Now Dumbass has a serious problem. If he goes to the

hospital with a gunshot wound, the police will be called, and then he'll have to explain he was trying to steal stuff from somebody and got shot. After he's treated, he'll be arrested and then, more than likely, be shipped off to jail again.

He decides to hide all day.

When night falls, Dumbass realizes he needs to get medical help or he's going to die. He makes his way to another house and knocks on the door. The man who answers sees a suspicious-looking man, sees the blood, and refuses to let Dumbass into the house. He agrees to call 911 but makes Dumbass wait down by the road until EMS comes and picks him up.

Dumbass is brought to a local hospital. They get to work stabilizing him and call for a helicopter to take him to a trauma hospital. Gunshot wounds often require a higher level of care than what's available in rural hospitals.

I get the call, and Eddie and I arrive with our equipment. A nurse who works there and knows us well sees us and literally bursts out laughing.

"What's up?" I ask. "What's so funny?"

She tells me Dumbass's story. Then we get serious because, once again, I'm about to walk into a situation where I have to deal with a white supremacist, one who is, in light of his prison record, possibly violent.

And I've got to fly him out of here.

When I walk into this man's room, nurses are working on him, trying to get another IV in him to give him blood. Dumbass is rolling around, pissed off that he got shot.

I see a swastika on his left temple. He got shot in his stomach, where he has a KKK tattoo and another one that says FUCK THE POLICE.

I just shake my head and start laughing.

Then I lean over and look right in Dumbass's face. I give him my biggest smile.

"What's up, man? I'm your nurse today. Your life is in my hands—no worries."

He doesn't say a word the entire flight.

I have no idea if the experiences these two men had with me changed them in any way. Quite frankly, it doesn't matter. I don't care what color you are. If I'm called to save your life, I'm going to do just that. You can thank me later.

DOMINIQUE SELBY

Dominique Selby grew up in Las Vegas. After graduating from high school, she enlisted in the navy as a hospital corpsman and worked in a clinic. She became one of the first women to go through the navy's rescue swimmer school. Dominique lives in Southern California and works full-time as a contractor with the navy's EMS director.

Y ou're going to a cancer floor," the U.S. Navy says.

I've just arrived at the San Diego Naval Medical Center, which treats veterans, service members, and their families. I graduated from nursing school, passed the NCLEX, and now have a nurse's license. I also have experience in search and rescue. I tell the navy I want to work in the emergency room.

"You're not going to the emergency room," the navy says. "You're going to be working in oncology."

I have no interest in oncology. The navy doesn't care. It puts you where it wants you or needs you, so I'm off to oncology.

I'm thinking I'm going to be serving an older population,

people who have lived a good life. It ends up being a lot of young people—and by *young*, I mean people in their twenties and thir-ties with really bad cancers like osteosarcomas, which attacks the bones and, more often than not, results in amputations.

One patient I have is twenty-six and suffering from brain cancer. He has one of those untreatable tumors. He lies in the dark by himself, and he's angry a lot of the time. His family is nowhere to be found. I don't know where or who they are or why they don't come visit him, but he ends up dying alone, by himself, in the dark.

It's horrible.

I've always been able to set my emotions aside when neces-sary. I don't know if that's good or bad, but it means I can approach my job very methodically and matter-of-factly.

I have a nineteen-year-old patient named Aaron who has been with us for months, maybe even a year. He's from Jamaica, the youngest of a bunch of kids, and he has an osteosarcoma. We've already cut off the lower part of his leg to try to get rid of the cancer. It keeps spreading up his leg, so we have to cut off part of his leg again—this time higher.

The cancer keeps spreading. We cut off half his pelvis, and then the cancer spreads into Aaron's abdomen, and at that point, there isn't anything we can do but put him in comfort care, which is basically hospice.

Aaron isn't ready to go and keeps crying for his mother. We can't get her to come over from Jamaica because she doesn't want to see her baby dying and in so much pain. It's a cultural thing, I'm sure, so we all hold his hand and try to give him medication to help the pain and just put him into that deep sleep.

Aaron keeps screaming, "I'm not ready to go! I don't want to die!"

It's so unnatural for me to be confronting the end of the life of a nineteen-year-old. It's unnatural as a health-care provider for me to just let someone go.

The way he dies, the whole experience—it's terrible. It breaks me. If I have to keep seeing these people, getting close to them and watching them die, it's going to drive me mad.

I walk over to my division chief.

"I'm done," I tell him. "I can't do this anymore."

I get transferred to Naval Hospital Camp Pendleton. I don't make it to the emergency room. I get placed into the ICU.

It's November of 2009. To get qualified as a critical-care nurse, I have to go through a lot of training. A few days into the new year, I work a night shift on Wednesday and come home early Thursday morning with the expectation of going back to work that night. When I wake up, I see I have all these missed calls from my superiors.

Did I do something wrong? Did I kill somebody? What's going on? I call my division officer.

"You know what's going on in the news, right?" she asks.

"You mean the earthquake in Haiti?"

"Yes. Don't come in tonight. We're going to send you to Haiti tomorrow or Saturday."

"For how long?"

"Plan on it being a regular six-month appointment."

Six *months?* The news is so sudden, so unexpected, I'm having a hard time comprehending what's happening.

Friday morning, my commissioning officer tells us we're

going to be a part of the surgical team taking in patients on one of the amphibious warships, the USS *Bataan*. It's designed to transport Marines, but the ship has huge medical capabilities.

Saturday, I'm on a plane with eighty other people. We get stuck in the Guantanamo Bay airport because the ship CEO didn't know we were all coming. He has no place to put us. While the navy tries to figure out logistics, we sleep on the floor of the airport.

When we arrive on the USS *Bataan,* we're all hoping to get some sleep. Instead, we get thirty-six incoming trauma patients. Helicopters have been scooping up injured people and dropping them on the ship.

It's chaos, an absolute shitshow. I'm told to head to the ICU.

Thirty-six incoming? How are we going to deal with that? I'm not prepared for this. I go into work mode and set all my feelings aside. I'm a master compartmentalizer.

The ICU is packed with people, many of whom are traumatically injured.

"What do you want me to do?" I ask one of the ICU guys.

"Just get to a bed and do something."

I'm brand-new in critical care, and I don't have any real training.

The doctors who came to the ship with me arrive at the ICU, and we start triaging, trying to figure out who needs to go to the OR right away and who can wait. There's so much going on I can barely pause to catch my breath.

All these patients are traumatically injured. We have to do amputations, and there's a language barrier. A rumor goes around Haiti: "Don't go to the Americans because they're going to cut off your arms and legs." The people are terrified of us. When I try to treat a young girl, she kicks me every time I get near her.

They put me on nights. Before I left for Haiti, my head nurse said, "There will be other nurses, ones with critical-care knowledge, who will help you. Bounce things off of them." But when I arrive for my shift, I don't have anyone else who is considered critical care—and I'm in charge of a fifteen-bed ICU on one side and a four-hundred-bed ward on the other.

It's a lot to deal with. And incredibly stressful.

I'm talking with another nurse who works in the ICU when a female corpsman from the ward side comes over to us and says, "Hey, I need a bag."

"What kind of bag?" I ask. "Like a trash bag?"

"No. Like a bag." The corpsman mimes squeezing a bag.

"You mean an Ambu bag?"

"Yes," she replies. "One of those. The lady next door stopped breathing."

I run over there, and sure enough, the lady isn't breathing.

I take charge. "Okay, we need to start breathing for her," I say. "Grab the gurney."

We bring the woman over to the ICU side and start running a code to resuscitate her. This is the first time I have to make major decisions on my own.

What am I going to do? Where is the doctor?

And we need a doctor. The problem is, the doctors aren't really assigned to any rooms, and we don't know where they are. I tell the corpsman, "Go and start knocking on doors and find one of the doctors."

The lady is breathing on her own when the doctor finally arrives. She's actually regaining consciousness.

Wow, I can actually do this. I trusted my calls. I was able to get through everything and direct people—and the woman is still alive. *This is awesome.*

Right after I get back from Haiti, I'm sent on a ten-month deployment to Afghanistan with the Marines as part of a mobile damage-control surgical team. The idea is, the patients come to us first. We're not there to fix them; we're there to find out where they're bleeding, stop the hemorrhaging, and then fly them to the next level of care. I'll be doing en route care by helicopter—the rotary medevacs used in theater.

My first helicopter flight is at night. The crew doesn't bring me any comms, so I'm unable to communicate with them while I'm basically by myself in the back of this 860, trying to resuscitate this patient who has lost his leg. Even with my ICU experience from working in Haiti, it's a very daunting task.

We have way too many patients. There aren't enough doctors and nurses to go around, so we're spread pretty thin. The burnout rate is high. A lot of the injury patterns are bilateral amputations, and a good majority of the young men I treat end up losing their genitals as well.

I try very hard not to hear a patient's name. I know that sounds cold, but if I get to know the patients, I have a hard time keeping them out of my head and end up thinking about them all the time. If I don't look at the patient as a person, I can focus on my job and help fix him.

The OR we work in doesn't have individual rooms. It's a six-bed open-bay OR, so you see everyone. The seemingly never-ending number of patients, the trauma and gore—it all gets to be overwhelming. *If one more kid comes in without his dick,* I tell myself, *I'm going to lose it.*

A British Marine team brings in a guy who has already lost one leg. The other one is badly mangled. When I see his penis, I breathe a sigh of relief. *Thank God, he still has his penis.*

A lot of times with these types of injuries, you have an ortho surgeon who is focusing on the extremities while a general surgeon focuses on the core—the abdomen and chest. I'm holding the soldier's leg that the ortho surgeon is cutting off when I see the general surgeon start amputating the soldier's penis.

I lose it. *"What are you doing?"*

The general surgeon shows me that the patient's boot had been blown off and the heel went into his abdomen and basically shredded the urethra and everything around it, leaving the surgeon no choice but to remove the penis.

The ortho surgeon finishes amputating the leg. I'm standing here, holding it in my hand, blood all over the floor and body parts sticking out everywhere I look, and for a moment I feel like I'm in the movie *Saw.*

Oh my God, this is insane. What am I doing?

Being thrown into all these different situations, the experience I gain from handling them, proves that I can do pretty much anything.

MEGAN OTTENBACHER

Megan Ottenbacher lives in Oklahoma and works as an ER nurse.

Growing up as the oldest sibling in my family, I'm a natural caretaker. I know I want to be either a teacher or a nurse.

I decide to try teaching first, and I'm the one who quickly learns a lesson. The best teachers have endless patience. I don't. I'd rather wipe grown men's butts for the rest of my life than take care of twenty-one kids every day. I quit my position as teacher's assistant and apply to work as a nurse's aide in the emergency room.

Hospitals have never, ever scared me. I've always been intrigued by them. My second week there, a guy in cardiac arrest is rushed into a room. I go about my business, leaving the heavy-duty stuff to the pros.

The unit secretary says to me, "You're going to do this one day, so you need to go in there and watch."

I go in and stand at the foot of the bed. The guy is fairly

young, and I'm handed his wallet. This is the time before smartphones, and a lot of people carry pictures in their wallets. I see a picture of him with a woman I'm assuming is his wife and a young boy around four years old.

That's when it hits me: This man is more than just a patient. He has a family.

I watch the doctors and nurses. They know their jobs and roles inside and out. After what feels like a long time, they get ROSC—a return of spontaneous circulation. Meaning they bring the man back and get a pulse.

And it's all because these doctors and nurses knew what to do, when to do it, and how to do it. Because of them, the woman and boy in the picture are going to have this man in their lives for that much longer. The wife is going to see her husband again, and the little boy still has his dad.

This moment solidifies my desire to be a nurse. I want to make a meaningful and lasting impact on people's lives.

When I graduate from nursing school, I apply for an externship at another local hospital. They offer me a position as a med-surg extern, which makes me mad because I applied to work in the ER.

"I want to work in the ER," I respectfully remind the hospital.

"I understand, but we don't have any spots. It's either this or, well, nothing."

I take the med-surg position.

It's the best thing that could have happened to me.

I learn how to manage six patients, medicate six patients, assess six patients, and interpret six different lab values for six different people. It teaches me everything I don't know about nursing and medicine.

One patient—a lady with an NG tube who is suffering from bowel pain—reshapes my professional life. This woman is a little on the needy side, but she's nice, so it's easier to put up with her when she's complaining. And she complains a lot.

"I'm hurting, I'm hurting," she says. "I'm in so much pain."

"Ma'am, I have given you everything I can possibly give you." I check my watch. "I can't give you anything else for another two hours. I'm sorry, but there's nothing more I can do."

I talk to another nurse about my patient.

"When did you do your last assessment?" the nurse asks.

"An hour, maybe more. I listened to her stomach. She was having pretty frequent bowel sounds."

"Let's reassess. Maybe something has changed."

We listen and discover that the woman doesn't have a single bowel sound in any quadrant. I know the reason even before the nurse says, "I think your patient has a bowel obstruction."

I take things very personally. I can't stop thinking that my patient is someone's mom—that I really could have hurt her if I hadn't conferred with that nurse.

Continual reassessment, I learn, is a vital part of any nursing field. It's always intervention, reassess, intervention, reassess. I can't just give meds or do some procedure and think it's going to fix the problem. As a nurse, you always have to reassess.

I don't come from a medical background. I don't have aunts or uncles who are in medicine. But each of my patients is someone's dad, brother, mother, sister, wife, husband. My job is to make sure they're comfortable. I treat them like I would want someone to treat my family.

When I go to work in the ICU, my thought is *I'm here to save people. I'm going to do everything I need to do to make sure these people return home.*

It's a very idealistic view of medicine.

I have patients well into their eighties who are on ventilators. Their families aren't ready to let them go. Some don't realize that their unconscious loved one coded and just had his or her ribs broken during CPR, that Grandma or Grandpa or whoever are never going to recover from the lifesaving measures we just gave them.

It's no quality of life—and it's not pretty.

Over time, I learn that maybe my part in saving people is letting them go.

"What would you do?" family members ask me.

My answer is always the same: "I really can't tell you what to do."

As an ICU nurse, you build a rapport with the families and they tend to trust you. While I can't give medical advice—that's the doctor's job—I can advise them on all the ways a situation can play out. That's how I can demonstrate my sympathy to their situation.

During my assessment with ICU patients, I ask them right up front what *they* would like done if medical intervention becomes necessary. You can't tiptoe around the question. In medicine, we can take extreme measures to prolong a patient's life, and a lot of patients don't want that.

This experience is the best preparation I could have as I move into working in the ER.

But I'm not emotionally prepared for it.

I'm doing CPR on a baby. The baby dies and then I have to go see another patient, a guy with an infected tooth. He's mad because it took me too long to get him his pain meds. What I don't understand yet—what a lot of people don't understand—is that as an ER nurse, you have to be able to switch gears fast.

I learn to compassionately compartmentalize. I try not to let tragedies enter my heart. I try to stay really present and in the moment. The emotional toll it takes on me is far greater than I realize.

My husband is a Marine who twice served in Iraq. When I come home and try to decompress, he says, "You don't know stress. You've never been to war."

"I understand that, but still, this is my experience, and I would really like to talk to you about it."

"You need to suck it up, Megan. You've never wiped someone's brains off your window."

Well, you know what? You've never held a dead baby. You've never had to give that dead baby to his mother. This is not a one-upping contest. I'm not trying to trade war stories with you. I'm just trying to let you know how hard my day was before I go feed our baby and then head off to soccer practice and coach all these little kids.

That's what I want to say. Instead, I bottle things up.

John, who is an ER nurse and an army veteran, is one of my good friends. We started out as ER techs together and maintained a close friendship even after I got married and moved away.

"Maybe you should start working out," he tells me.

It's a good idea. I'm still carrying extra weight from nursing school and from having a baby.

I start going to the gym. I meet up with John and do a couple of half-marathons with him, and I talk to him about my life and my marriage. I attend church and see a marriage counselor.

These things help, but my workdays still feel like I'm running a marathon. I go, go, go until I crash. I cry, then I pick myself up and start the marathon all over again.

My new job involves working Air Evac. We get a call about a massive motor-vehicle collision on a major interstate. I'm fairly new to this role, but I'm partnered with a super-knowledgeable paramedic named Henry who is simply awesome.

"Chances are we're going to have to intubate the patient," he tells me as we're in flight on a rinky-dink Bell 206. "We're probably going to see some burns."

He's running me through some mental drills when there's talk over our headset: "Air Evac 83, please be advised that Air Evac 36 is en route."

A moment later, we receive word that two additional helicopters are also in the air. There are now going to be four birds responding to a collision on a major highway.

"We're going to circle around," our pilot tells us. "EMS is going to triage and let us know who needs to fly down first."

Seeing four helicopters circling around the accident, listening to the comms from four different pilots as we wait to be dispatched to the ground—it's like a scene out of a movie. Listening to the pilots communicating reminds me of the camaraderie we all share, that we're brothers and sisters here to do a very important job.

We're the second bird to land. I grab the blood and equipment, and then Henry and I are off and running.

Henry kneels next to the head of the patient. I kneel by the foot. The patient is male, thirty-four, not much older than me, and has a broken femur and a flail chest—severe blunt-force trauma has caused several ribs to separate from his rib cage. He has a collapsed lung, and he's working very hard to breathe.

There are seven cars piled up behind us, and the helicopters are generating so much noise that it's impossible to hear each other. But we don't need to talk. Henry and I make eye contact, and we know exactly what each one of us has to do, and we do it without speaking a single word.

We get our patient loaded onto the helicopter. His name is Alex, and as I'm administering medications—paralytics and sedatives—he looks up at us and says, gasping, "Please don't let me die. Please don't let me die."

"Honey," I say, grabbing his hand, "we've got you. Don't you worry."

The meds put Alex to sleep. Henry intubates him.

Our pilot is booking it. We arrive at the hospital in fifteen minutes. My arms, the cot—everything is covered in blood.

Shortly thereafter, I hear that there was a fatality in the crash. My thoughts turn to Alex. I call the ICU to check on him.

"He's stable," the nurse tells me. "His wife just walked in the door about thirty minutes ago."

I feel a flood of emotion. A wife has her husband because of what we did today. It's the pinnacle of my career.

A week later, I'm doing some training in Tulsa. I'm wearing

my Air Evac uniform and Alex is still weighing on my mind. His is the first legit trauma case I've experienced outside of a hospital setting, and since he's recuperating in a hospital close by, I decide to visit.

When I arrive, Alex is sitting up in bed, talking to his wife and his parents. They hug me and, choking back tears, keep saying, "Thank you. Thank you so much."

"I didn't do it by myself," I say. "I had a great medic and a pilot who flew like hell."

Alex swallows. "My friend riding in the car with me that day." He takes a deep breath, steadies himself. "He died."

"I'm so sorry for that," I say. "I truly am. But look around you. Your wife is here. Your mom and dad are here. Be thankful that they don't have to deal with what your friend's family is going through right now."

"I know," he says, resigned but grateful. "I know."

When I started out as a nurse's aide, I wanted to be a person who made a difference in someone's life. Now, seven years later, I am that person.

TENEILLE TAYLOR

Growing up in Herndon, Virginia, Teneille Taylor was so driven to take care of people that everyone called her "the love bug." The OR externship she did during her senior year in nursing school made her fall in love with surgery. Teneille is a flight nurse for PHI Air Medical, a medevac air-ambulance service in Virginia.

My first year of nursing, I worked in the operating room as a scrub/circulator nurse, handing equipment to the surgeons and taking care of patients perioperatively.

All my life I've been looking inside medical books at these neat cartoon-like depictions of spleens, stomachs, intestines—even brains. Seeing organs in real life is completely different. They're covered in blood and fat and everything else; it doesn't look remotely like any of those pictures in textbooks.

I know it sounds crazy, but it's awesome to touch something that's warm and slippery. *This is the coolest thing.*

As much as I love my job, it's very intimidating. A lot of yelling goes on in the OR. Some surgeons aren't super-friendly, and some just scream and yell because it's their personality.

I'm a type A personality, but I'm also very tenderhearted. If I get yelled at, I start crying—not because I'm upset or mad but because I can't control that emotion. I find it hard to toughen myself up in such a stressful environment.

One surgery involved amputating the leg of an ICU patient. After surgery, I'm told to bring it to the morgue.

Carrying a leg wrapped in a red biohazard bag at three a.m. on a Saturday, the halls virtually empty, is a surreal experience. As I walk, my thoughts return to a disconnect I've been experiencing for a while now.

As much as I love being in the OR, in terms of patient care, it's very hands-off. I want to do real, hands-on nursing.

When I reach the morgue, I don't see anyone. I put the leg on the desk and leave.

When I return to work on Monday, a coworker says, "You left a leg in the morgue."

"Yeah, that's where I was told to put it."

He looks at me as though I've lost my mind. "That leg rotted over the weekend. It putrefied. They're having to air out the morgue right now. Do you have any idea what that smelled like?"

I get defensive. "I was told to put it in the morgue. I don't know what else you thought I should have—"

"Why didn't you put it in one of the drawers?" He's beside himself.

"I've never been to the morgue before," I say. "And it's not as though there was a call bell like when you go to an apartment to, you know, ring somebody. Even if I knew where the drawers were, I wasn't going to go opening random drawers and just stick a leg in there. That's crazy."

The news about the leg is all over the hospital. I've caused a big stir.

Soon after, I decide it's time to leave the OR and try to get into ICU nursing.

I get an interview for the adult special-care unit at a hospital in Virginia. They hire me because I have a year of nursing experience.

The OR, I quickly discover, exists in a totally different world than the rest of the hospital. My preceptor is irritated with me because I don't know simple, basic procedures, like how to hang a new IV bag.

They don't teach you that at nursing school. You learn about acronyms and body systems. You do some practice stuff, like putting an NG tube or an IV in a mannequin, but I've never done either one on an actual person.

It's like I'm starting from scratch.

And it's pretty rough, because the people here are critically ill. The learning curve is steep. I've inherited my mom's looks and nice skin, so although I'm twenty-two, I look much, much younger.

"Are you old enough to be a nurse?" my patients keep asking me.

I work nights, which is difficult because I'm not a night owl. Even after nine hours of sleep in my bed at home, I wake up feeling nauseated, my head pounding like I have the flu. But the night people are amazing. There's a big difference between day babes—the day nurses—and the night shift. The night-crew people are cool and fun. There is a huge sense of teamwork. There's no management or anyone breathing down your neck.

In 2005, we get a twenty-two-year-old patient who was involved in a DUI. His name is Jeffrey Fearnow. He'd been drinking and driving on a back road, crashed, and was ejected from his truck.

Jeffrey is rushed into the trauma bay and given a whole-body CT scan. He has a lacerated spleen, a cracked skull, broken ribs, a fractured collarbone, and a traumatic brain injury. His brain is bleeding and swelling.

To relieve the intracranial pressure, he undergoes an emergency bilateral craniotomy: two sections of his skull are temporarily removed to allow his brain to swell in response to the injury.

Bone flaps—the pieces of skull—are stored via one of two methods: cryopreservation in a freezer set at a subzero temperature or in abdominal subcutaneous pockets, which is a safer method, as there is less chance for the bones to grow bacteria. Because of the severity of Jeffrey's trauma, his bone flaps are stored in a freezer. While he's healing, he will have to wear a special helmet, given that large areas of his brain will be covered only with skin and tissue.

He's placed in a medically induced coma so he can heal. He spends nearly four weeks in the ICU. After his sedation is weaned, he awakens and is alert and able to follow commands and protect his own airway without the breathing tube. The doctors decide Jeffrey is well enough to be discharged to a rehabilitation center. He requires a rehab facility because his muscles have atrophied while he has been in the hospital. Rehabilitation is structured like a school day. He undergoes physical and occupational therapy every day. He learns to walk, stand, and sit up on his own. He has to relearn coordination, how to swallow and eat—all while wearing the helmet to protect his brain.

Jeffrey is young and pissed off at the world, at the situation he finds himself in, at the fact that he has to be at rehab with old people and wear this helmet, which he feels makes him look like a freak. After completing rehab and being discharged home, he is a groomsman in a friend's wedding. He refuses to wear his helmet because he doesn't want people staring at him, but people stare anyway because his skull is clearly misshapen from the surgery.

The day comes when the bone flaps can be reattached to his skull. He undergoes surgery. When he wakes up in the PACU—the post-anesthesia care unit—he sees his mother, who has been constantly by his side, and for the first time the extent of what he's put her through these past few months hits him. Instead of being angry, he's contrite.

"I'm really, really sorry, Mom." He knows the pain and grief his drinking-and-driving accident caused her. "Thanks for being here."

Jeffrey is moved to the neuro ICU. He's complaining of headaches, which isn't abnormal now that his brain is back in a tight, enclosed space. Over the next twenty-four hours, we do one-hour checks—seeing if he can hold a conversation, taking a look at his pupils, waking him up at night.

By midafternoon the following day, Jeffrey has become nonresponsive. He shows no reaction when we poke his collarbone or pinch the inside of his leg. He doesn't move his hand away when we push a pin on a nail bed. He's given an emergency CT scan.

His brain is bleeding and swelling again. Doctors also see signs of infection. Jeffrey undergoes another bilateral craniotomy. Both bone flaps are removed, and because of the infection, they can never go back in. In the future, he'll need custom prosthetic bone flaps.

After that surgery and emergent re-removal of his bone flaps, Jeffrey is permanently comatose. His eyes are open, but no one is home.

Weeks turn into months, and Jeffrey is still with us.

His healthy body has withered to skin and bones. We can see his hip bones sticking out, and he's knobby and contracted—his arms pulling up toward his chest, his knees drawn up.

Jeffrey's family—his mom, Jan; his stepdad, Pepper; and his sister, Jackie—are constantly at his bedside. Jan works from his hospital room.

All the nurses, me especially, become very attached to Jeffrey and his family. We make sure Jeffrey is always ready for them—deodorant, a brand-new gown, freshly shaven, mouth cleaned, whatever he needs. On his birthday, I put a little hat on him—the giant clownfish from *Finding Nemo*.

When his mom walks into his room, we hear her mock-yell, "Oh, Jeffrey, what have they done to you?"

Jeffrey is with us for seven months. During that time, he undergoes multiple surgeries and suffers more complications. He contracts pneumonia and MRSA. His spinal fluid isn't draining correctly. He has several abdominal surgeries for various obstructions. He's on a feeding tube and will be for the rest of his life.

It's now 2006. Doctors tell Jan, his mother, that it's time to place him in a nursing home. Finding a nursing facility proves difficult. There aren't many options available, so Jan decides to take her son home. She has a hospital bed set up in their living room. She's also purchased a crucial piece of equipment: a standing platform. It will lift Jeffrey and keep him upright to help fluid drain from his lungs. She fights for in-home physical therapy and anything else she can get to benefit Jeffrey.

Jan calls me one day to ask a favor. "Jeffrey's stepbrother is getting married in a couple of weeks. Would you be willing to, well, babysit Jeffrey while we're at the wedding?"

"Absolutely." Jeffrey and his family are a big part of my career and an even bigger part of my heart.

While they're at the wedding, I take care of Jeffrey—turn him over, change his diapers, monitor his feeding tube. I visit the family several other times to say hello. I see them at Christmas.

The following year, I'm in Europe with friends when I have a vivid dream in which Jeffrey wakes up. My friends know about Jeffrey, his story, and I tell them all about my dream because it felt so incredibly real. I'm traveling, so I don't think to reach out to Jan.

In spring of 2009, Jan is outside working in her garden when she hears Jeffrey call, "Mom."

She drops her tools and, her heart bursting with joy, rushes into the house.

Her son lies in his bed, unresponsive. He's not on a ventilator because you can't be on a ventilator long term, and technically, his lungs work; he has a tube inserted in his trachea that can be suctioned to remove secretions from his lungs.

"Did you just call for me?" Jan asks. She stares at his lips, expecting them to move.

Jeffrey stares at her. He doesn't speak. He's been home with her now for two and a half years. All that time he has been completely silent.

Soon after, I text Jan to check in on her and Jeffrey. I also share the dream I had on vacation about her son waking up.

Jan texts back that she'd thought Jeffrey had called her. She tells me she's sure she imagined it because when she ran back inside the house, she saw that vacant look in his eyes and was reminded that there was no possible way he could have spoken.

One evening in May, Jan sits down at her son's bed, like she does every night, and says, "You know what, Jeffrey? Tomorrow is Mother's Day. It would be really nice if you could just say my name or say hi to me."

"Uh-huh," he mumbles. His voice is so whisper-quiet because of disuse that she wonders if she imagined it. But she knows she didn't. She *heard* him. She was sitting right here and heard her son speak.

This is real, this is happening.

Jan bursts into tears.

Jan takes Jeffrey to his regular checkups with his neurosurgeon and other doctors. She tells them that her son spoke to her. They're not dismissive, but they're not encouraging either. They tell her not to get her hopes up.

By Father's Day, Jeffrey is alert and starting to speak. Pepper leans down, bringing his ear close to Jeffrey's mouth, and says, "I heard you say something. What did you say?"

Jeffrey's voice is incredibly weak, but Pepper can make out the words: "Happy Father's Day."

Other people come in to talk to Jeffrey, and soon he can remember their names after they've left. He asks about the dogs, knows their names.

The neurologists can't believe it. Can't explain it.

I'm on shift a few weeks later when Jan brings Jeffrey to visit the hospital.

I just about hit the floor. Everyone does. Every single one of us bursts into tears of joy because we can't believe what we're witnessing.

Jeffrey is in a wheelchair, but he can use a walker. He's put on weight. He can talk, but his speech is slow, the words slurred. He doesn't know who I am—he doesn't remember any of us.

"Jeffrey," his mom says, "this is Teneille, one of the nurses who took such great care of you."

I give him a hug and a kiss. Seeing him up and walking, using his arms and legs, hearing him talk—it's the best feeling I've experienced in my life. His recovery is truly a miracle. It will take a long time for him to relearn the hundreds of daily tasks most of us take for granted—how to feed himself, how to wash his hair—but he keeps working toward recovery.

Jeffrey now lives with his girlfriend and her son.

He can drive a car. He speaks to school-age kids about his accident. He has almost completely recovered.

And now I'm a flight nurse on a helicopter. I've dealt with

all kinds of crazy trauma, done all sorts of crazy medical procedures, like drilling into people's bones and putting needles in their chests. I've volunteered for medical missions and traveled all over the world, gone to places like villages in Vietnam and Haiti, where I've given primary care, checking blood pressure and blood sugars and handing out vitamins to people who are shockingly poor and hungry. I've seen a lot of people die.

Jeffrey is never far from my mind.

I think a lot about the families of my patients. The time I've spent with them—sometimes weeks and months, sometimes nowhere near that long. There are many hundreds of families I've put my arms around in joy and despair. My job isn't just taking care of patients. I take care of families too.

It's the greatest gift.

PART FOUR:

Thank You

SHANNON MILLER

Shannon Miller grew up in a small farm town about seventy miles from Detroit, Michigan. She graduated from nursing school in 2001 and has worked in the ER, cath lab, and most of the surgical suites. Shannon lives in Royal Oak, Michigan, where she works as a registered nurse in surgical services.

As a nurse, you've got to have your best day on someone else's worst day.

It's a beautiful summer day in Metro Detroit. A family is out tubing on one of the city's busier inner lakes. The dad is piloting a Jet Ski and pulling a tube holding his eleven-year-old son and two daughters, ages six and ten.

But he's not using a "spotter"—a boating term for the person who keeps an eye on everyone and alerts the driver if someone falls into the water. The dad is cruising along, enjoying the summer day and the laughter of his kids, unaware of the boat approaching from behind at a rapid speed.

The boat hits his kids.

The children are rushed to a nearby hospital that's staffed to handle pediatric trauma. The boy passes away. The two girls are transported less than ten miles to my hospital. We hear they're coming and prep the trauma room for their arrival.

The two girls...their bodies are okay, just some scrapes and scratches, but their skulls are crushed. They don't look like kids. They don't look like anything.

It makes me want to cry—but I can't. I have to go into work mode.

Okay, I tell myself. *Here we go.*

The family is large, and the hospital staff puts them all in a conference room. This makeshift waiting area is maybe two hundred feet from the trauma room where we're working on the girls, trying to save their lives. Through the walls, we can hear the family's bloodcurdling screams, the kind that hurt your soul.

Before coming to the ICU, I worked mainly as a cardiac nurse. My patients were older—men and women who had lived good, long lives. Death was expected, the natural way of things.

But this—this is my first time witnessing such severe trauma. I go into a functional state of shock. I'm working, performing my duties, but I can't believe what I'm seeing.

The six-year-old makes it out of the trauma bay and goes to the OR. The other girl—the one I'm working with, the ten-year-old—seems to be responding to painful stimuli. When we perform a sternal rub, closing a fist and vigorously using the knuckles, she reacts in ways that give us hope.

A pediatric neurosurgeon has reviewed the CT scan, and he

swoops into the trauma room like Batman to insert a tube to reduce the swelling in her brain. He immediately starts drilling into her head without anesthesia—without anything.

I never expected so see this in a suburban trauma center.

There is no chance this girl's going to live. There's just no hope. This is what you do when your bag of tricks is empty. This is all we have left.

Over the years, I've learned to treat my patients as files in my mental filing cabinet. When someone dies, I take him or her, all of my emotions—every single one that accompanies that particular event—and place them into a file. Then I tuck the file in the cabinet, shut the door, and move on so I can be the best for the next person who needs my help.

I decompress when I go home. I'll cry and relive the wails of the family, the terrified looks on their faces, their heartache and grief, and feel absolutely rotten for a few days because I couldn't help them.

The six-year-old who was rushed into surgery ends up passing away. The ten-year-old I helped treat is in the pediatric ICU. She's going to be here at the hospital for some time, and every once in a while, I ask someone in the PICU how the girl is doing.

"She's doing okay," I'm usually told. "Not great, but there are signs of improvement."

My significant other is a child psychologist. I can talk to him about my feelings, but he doesn't want to hear the gory medical details, the blood and guts.

The things nurses see—people don't know how we deal with it, how we compartmentalize it. We need people in our own field that we can talk to, vent to. Having a sisterhood—or brotherhood, in the case of guy nurses—acts as a kind of therapy.

I get a male patient at the ER. He's sitting in a chair, and I'm taking his vitals when I ask, "What brings you into the hospital today?"

He looks at me dead straight. His expression reminds me of an incident where a male psych patient whipped a telephone at my head. *Your full name is printed on your badge,* he said to me. *I will find where you live, and I will come kill you.* After that, I applied for a weapon and eventually got one so I could protect myself at home.

The man sitting in the chair says, "The bitch done got me."

My heart is racing. This guy strikes me as someone who could potentially turn violent.

"Could you give me some more information?" I ask. "Are you hurt? Were you assaulted?"

He spreads his legs out, points to his crotch, and says, "The bitch done got me."

"Did something happen to your genitals?"

"Yeah, she got me. That bitch, she done got me."

"Do you think you may have contracted something from a female partner?"

"Yes, that's it. She's a bitch. She didn't tell me she was all skanky."

You can't make this stuff up. "All righty," I say. "Well, let's get you checked out."

Needless to say, I find out he wasn't using condoms.

One of the regular visitors to the ER is a woman who has cancer and is on chemo. She gets really dehydrated, which is common when you're on chemo, and not everyone in the ER knows how to access a mediport, a flexible tube that's placed under the skin in a vein in a patient's chest, allowing nurses to take blood and give IV medication and fluids.

A nurse asks me if I can help. I do and end up meeting the woman's three daughters. We get their mother hydrated and send her up to the floor.

"We come in a lot," one of the daughters says to me. "Not everybody, obviously, can help her. Next time we come in, can we ask for you?"

"Sure. Absolutely."

I see this woman and her daughters quite a few times over the next several months. They're all very nice people. The daughters share how their mom is doing. The woman doesn't look well, but I can tell she's fighting to stay alive.

I'm at a grocery store when I see one of the woman's daughters. Seeing her makes me think about their mother. I haven't seen her come into the ER for hydration in quite a while. I try to think positive thoughts. Sometimes with cancer, positive outcomes can happen.

The daughter comes to me and says, "You're the one who helped my mom with her port."

I nod. "At the ER."

"You were never too busy for us. You always sat and talked to us and treated us nice, like we're human beings."

"How is your mom?"

"She passed away," the daughter replies.

"I'm sorry. I'm so, so sorry."

The woman sees the pained expression on my face and says, "I don't want you to be sad about it. I came to talk to you because I want you to feel good about what you did. We all appreciated how you helped her. It meant a lot to my mom that you would sit and talk to her—talk to us—and just be nice, because a lot of people in the ER are just so rushed. You made such an impact on us, and I wanted you to know that. And to thank you."

Her words made me feel six feet tall. Bulletproof. More often than not, I don't know what happens to patients after they leave the ER. You don't necessarily get any follow-ups.

Six months later, I'm at home watching the news and see a report on the ten-year-old girl whose siblings were killed in the boating accident. She has returned to school after months of physical and occupational therapy. She looks like a normal kid and seems to be acting like a normal kid with her friends.

That's a good feeling, to actually see how I helped someone recover. The family had a horrible, horrible situation, but to see that one child make it out alive—to me, that's a miracle. It's truly a miracle because I saw what she looked like when she came into the trauma room.

CLAIRE

Claire has been an ER nurse for nine years. She works at an inner-city hospital.

I'm working the night shift, checking the vitals on a patient, when I hear a lady moaning in the hallway—the kind of moan that immediately signals something isn't right.

I poke my head out of the room and see one of our paramedics with our triage nurse, who is pushing a pregnant lady in a wheelchair. The triage nurse sees me and says, "I'm bringing this woman up to labor and delivery."

The pregnant woman moans again. "We're not going to make it upstairs."

The triage nurse wheels her into one of our code rooms. The medic and I follow.

The woman is wearing a dress. Before the paramedic and triage nurse lift the woman to her feet, I look between her legs and see that, for some reason, she's not wearing any underwear.

I also see the baby presenting.

The umbilical cord is wrapped twice around the infant's neck. I'm the only one wearing gloves. As I'm unwrapping the cord, they lift the woman up onto the bed, and the baby literally falls into my hands.

This is pretty cool, I think. I've been a nurse for only six months.

They say you learn a lot of things when you're in nursing school, but you know nothing when you get out.

It's true. When I first start, I'm completely overwhelmed. One of the nursing supervisors gives me some great advice: "Remember, you can do *anything* for twelve hours."

The young girl who comes into the ER is nineteen. Her name is Tina, and she's accompanied by her mother and a friend.

Tina looks distraught. In a voice stripped of emotion, she explains that she and her friends were out drinking and smoked some marijuana. "My friends decided they wanted to leave the party," Tina continues. "I decided to stay. When I was ready to go, I called an Uber."

"Where was this?" I ask.

Tina gives me the address. I know the area. It's downtown, not the best neighborhood.

Tina takes a deep breath to steady herself. Swallows. The mother, her eyes puffy and bloodshot, rubs her daughter's back while Tina's friend stares at the floor, crying silently. Horrified.

"There was this guy outside, where I was waiting for my Uber," Tina says, her voice shaky. "I asked him for a cigarette."

Then her voice breaks. "He pulled me behind a building and he ... he ..."

She can't say the word; she bursts into tears.

The mother says, "She was a virgin."

My heart aches for this young woman.

Our hospital has a twenty-four-hour SANE (Sexual Assault Nurse Examiners) unit—a safe space that collects forensic evidence and provides medical care to victims of sexual assault.

I take Tina and hand her off to our SANE nurses and doctor. I'm not present for the exam, always performed by a nurse, but I'm asked to take the girl's urine sample to the lab. The semen is visible to the naked eye.

After I drop off the sample, I check in with my other patients, many of whom are frustrated. I can't say I kept them waiting because I was tied up with someone who was raped. On other days, I'm delayed with someone who just lost a parent or whose child just died of a drug overdose.

We get another young patient, a man who jumped off the ninth floor of a hotel. The police arrived first, and they ended up doing CPR. The young man is severely disfigured—legs broken, big lacerations. He's pretty much dead on arrival.

Later, I find out he had cerebral palsy. He left a suicide note.

As an ER nurse, you learn very quickly to keep your emotions in check. Any nurse who doesn't ends up in an endless pit of depression.

I'm too busy between school and work to have time for a lot of hobbies, but I make time for CrossFit-style workouts. A lot of nurses, firefighters, and police officers seem to gravitate to CrossFit because the fitness regimen really clears the mind.

My boyfriend is in the navy, and I'm taking care of his dog, Ranger, while he's deployed overseas. Ranger also helps me cope on the rough days.

When I return to work, a lady in her forties is admitted with end-stage cancer. She's accompanied to the hospital by her mother. I feel so incredibly bad for her—no parent should ever have to bury a child.

The mom is crying. There's not much anyone can say in a situation like this, but I try to be there as much as I can.

As we're bringing the cancer patient upstairs to a room, the mom gives me a hug. Normally, I don't like being touched at work, but this woman has endeared herself to me.

"Thank you so much," the mom says.

She's the one dealing with this incredible burden, and here she is thanking me.

I think about the man who committed suicide and the young woman who was brutally raped; of the patients who have died. Dealing with loss and tragedy day after day—I know it won't get any easier no matter how long I do this work. There will always be cases that will get to me because this is an emotional job.

But this woman who just thanked me—it's moments like these that make me and other nurses do what we do. We all want to make a difference for someone who needs it.

JODY A. JAMIESON-LIANA

Jody A. Jamieson-Liana grew up in Marquette, Michigan. An ER nurse like her mom, she also teaches cardiac life support at a hospital in Wisconsin.

My patient is a single mother named Sandy who is suffering from headaches severe enough to affect her vision.

"They've been bad for a while," she tells me. "But I had to change jobs, and my insurance isn't the best, so..."

I see this a lot, people putting off medical care due to the limitations of their insurance. And now, because of COVID, even more people are staying home.

As I'm examining her, Sandy starts telling me about her life. She talks about her work and about her daughter, who is now ten. Before her daughter was born, Sandy worked with animals, and then she became a nanny, a job she loves because she has such a positive impact on families. Now, because of COVID, she's at home with her kid.

"We should probably do an MRI," I tell her. I'm hoping Sandy is suffering from a migraine and not, worst-case scenario, a brain tumor.

Her MRI is horrible. She has a mass so big, it has shifted part of her brain.

"You're going to need brain surgery," the doctor tells her.

"When?"

"Like, tomorrow."

I'm watching Sandy trying to process everything. I'm a mother, and I know she's thinking about her child right now.

"Okay," Sandy says, her voice emotionless because she's in shock. "All right. I...I'm not sure what I'm going to do. I don't have any family in the area, and I have to have someone watch my daughter. Then there's the money for the surgery. I don't know how I'm going to pay for that."

Later, I'm still thinking about Sandy. The bill for this surgery is going to be hanging over her head for the next fifteen or so years. She'll always be behind on her payments.

I decide to go speak to my manager, Denise. She's a beautiful soul and one of the strongest leaders at our hospital.

"We really need to do something for this woman," I say after explaining Sandy's situation. "Would you be okay if we set up a GoFundMe page to help pay for her surgery?"

The rules for hospitals advocating for patients vary from state to state. There's also a lot of red tape. But if there's anyone who can pull this off, it's Denise.

"Absolutely," Denise says. "We need to do something for her."

Helping patients always feels good, but Sandy is one of my fondest memories. She is such a positive person throughout her medical procedures, and no matter how she's feeling, no matter how much pain or discomfort she's in, she always greets us with a smile.

I remember my patients through their smiles. The thank-yous.

Thank you for being here with me. Thank you for holding my hand. Thank you for looking into my eyes and telling me everything is going to be okay.

MICHELLE RYLANDER

Michelle Rylander majored in premed and then chose nursing for flexibility and life balance during motherhood. She lives in Plano, Texas, and has worked as a pediatric nurse practitioner for nearly three decades.

I love being able to take care of people's kids.

Every morning, I pray for opportunity. I ask God to allow me to be a blessing to the people I encounter, especially my patients and their families.

I work in a children's hospital but, fortunately, not in an ICU. I see children get sick and undergo surgery, and while they may be unwell for a time, the good majority of them get better.

Sick babies are so pitiable because you can't console them or explain to them that the medicine will make them feel better. Even young kids, they hate you when you have to give them shots, put in an IV—anything that's painful—but they get better so much quicker than any other age group. The younger the child, the better the prospects for healing.

The girl who is having elective surgery today for a hernia repair is beautiful and healthy. Because anesthesia can suppress breathing, she's put on a ventilator during surgery.

I'm shocked when she starts to code—she doesn't have a heartbeat adequate to sustain life. We need to correct the little girl's heart rhythm right away or she'll die.

The anesthesiologist delivers medication that, combined with CPR, will facilitate resuscitation. One of the two surgeons in the operating room starts chest compressions.

We get a heartbeat back on the monitor.

I feel a surge of joy.

"We're losing her again," the surgeon says.

Someone else takes over chest compressions. We get a heartbeat again and feel another surge of hope. Then the heartbeat disappears again.

And again.

And again.

Adrenaline is a powerful hormone, but performing good-quality chest compressions is fatiguing, which is why we take turns doing CPR. Other medical staff gown up and come in to assist. In a situation like this, it's all hands on deck.

I've got this, I tell myself as I wait for my turn. This little girl is counting on me—my coworkers are counting on me. I so badly want to be able to do the right thing.

For the next forty-five minutes, we see glimmers of hope—the heartbeat coming back because the medications are kicking in—only to have that hope ripped away.

It's become evident that she's not going to survive.

"We need to bring her mother in here," the surgeon says.

Parents have a difficult time accepting a healthy child's sudden death. In an emergency setting like this, you want the family to be able to see all the effort that is being made to save their child—that *everything* that can possibly be done is, in fact, being done.

You also want the family to have a moment to speak to their son or daughter before the heartbeat is gone. To give the mom, dad, and siblings a chance to express and show love.

I'm doing chest compressions when the mother and the girl's sister are brought into the OR. The mother wails. I can't see the girl's sister because there are so many people in the room and because I'm focused on performing CPR.

Sometime later, while we're all still working on the girl, a nurse ushers the mother and daughter out of the OR to try to answer their questions and offer comfort.

I don't know what it's like resuscitating an adult, but people have a really hard time stopping CPR on a child. We will go and go.

And we do. We keep doing chest compressions for another thirty or so minutes.

The physician in charge says, "That's enough."

He calls it.

We're devastated. For the past hour and a half, we worked so hard on trying to resuscitate this sweet young girl.

Later that night, I'm still thinking about the mother. The sounds she made. She came into the hospital with her healthy daughter for a routine operation, and she left without her daughter.

None of the terrible things that happen are a surprise to

God. He knows what the day will bring, and I know He will test me. My compassion, sympathy, and empathy are gifts from God, and knowing I've done my very best to do His work helps.

There are days when I find I can't shut down my thoughts and feelings. On these days, I have a glass or two of wine. It doesn't fix the problem, but it does help mute my thoughts and feelings for a little bit.

I drink a lot of wine that night.

I have so many wonderful memories from working in pediatrics. I've felt the sweet hugs from babies and young kids and seen the looks on their faces. I've seen conjoined twins separated to a beautiful outcome. I've had a family name their baby after me, which was incredible and too kind.

My favorite memory is when I was a baby nurse, straight out of school. That first year, I'm given the night shift and some holidays. The month of December, I'm that person who wears holiday-appropriate clothing and jewelry every single day. The window-washers are dressed up like superheroes. You can get away with things like that when you work at a children's hospital.

It's late on Christmas Eve, and everyone on the floor is asleep. The only sound I hear is a Midnight Mass quietly playing on a family TV in one of the rooms.

I turn my attention to the brand-new stuffed animals that were donated to the hospital.

We were supposed to hand them out to the patients on Christmas Day, but I said, "Oh, no, please let me hand them out when the children are asleep."

I feel like Santa as I go around the floor putting these little stuffed animals into cribs and beds where sleeping children will wake and discover the gifts on Christmas morning.

I finish my rounds well past midnight then go directly to my parents' home, where we'll celebrate Christmas together. Later in the day, we turn on the news, and I'm surprised to see a story about my hospital. Someone found out that stuffed animals were placed in the children's beds while they slept, and the reporter is interviewing families.

"It was so magical," a grateful mother says. "My son woke up and thought Santa had come."

Watching the parents, seeing the joy on their faces and on the faces of their children—it's such a sweet surprise.

ABOUT THE AUTHORS

James Patterson is the world's bestselling author and most trusted storyteller. He has created many enduring fictional characters and series, including Alex Cross, the Women's Murder Club, Michael Bennett, Maximum Ride, Middle School, and I Funny. Among his notable literary collaborations are *The President Is Missing,* with President Bill Clinton, and the Max Einstein series, produced in partnership with the Albert Einstein estate. Patterson's writing career is characterized by a single mission: to prove that there is no such thing as a person who "doesn't like to read," only people who haven't found the right book. He's given over three million books to schoolkids and the military, donated more than seventy million dollars to support education, and endowed over five thousand college scholarships for teachers. For his prodigious imagination and championship of literacy in America, Patterson was awarded the 2019 National Humanities Medal. The National Book Foundation presented him with the Literarian Award for

Outstanding Service to the American Literary Community, and he is also the recipient of an Edgar Award and nine Emmy Awards. He lives in Florida with his family.

Matt Eversmann retired from the army after twenty years of service. His first book with James Patterson was *Walk in My Combat Boots*.

Chris Mooney is the international bestselling author of fourteen thrillers. The Mystery Writers of America nominated *Remembering Sarah* for an Edgar Award. He teaches creative writing at Harvard.

For a complete list of books by

JAMES PATTERSON

VISIT
JamesPatterson.com

 Follow James Patterson on Facebook
@JamesPatterson

 Follow James Patterson on Twitter
@JP_Books

 Follow James Patterson on Instagram
@jamespattersonbooks